BioEngagement

A Horizon in Bioethics Series Book from

THE CENTER FOR
BIOETHICS
AND HUMAN DIGNITY

The Horizons in Bioethics Series brings together an array of insightful writers to address important bioethical issues from a forward-looking Christian perspective. The introductory volume, *Bioethics and the Future of Medicine*, covers a broad range of topics and foundational matters. Subsequent volumes focus on a particular set of issues, beginning with the end-of-life theme of *Dignity and Dying* and continuing with the genetics focus of *Genetic Ethics*, the economic and patient-caregiver emphases of *The Changing Face of Health Care*, and the reproductive and sexuality topics of *The Reproductive Revolution*.

The series is a project of The Center for Bioethics and Human Dignity, an international center located just north of Chicago, Illinois, in the United States of America. The Center endeavors to bring Christian perspectives to bear on today's many pressing bioethical challenges. It pursues this task by developing two book series, six audio tape series, six video tape series, numerous conferences in different parts of the world, and a variety of other printed and computer-based resources. Through its membership program, the Center networks and provides resources for people interested in bioethical matters all over the world. Members receive the Center's international journal, *Ethics and Medicine*, the Center's newsletter, *Dignity*, the Center's Update Letters, special World Wide Web access, an Internet News Service and Discussion Forum, and discounts on a wide array of bioethics resources.

For more information on membership in the Center or its various resources, including present or future books in the Horizons in Bioethics Series, contact the Center at:

The Center for Bioethics and Human Dignity
2065 Half Day Road
Bannockburn, IL 60015 USA
Phone: (847) 317-8180
Fax: (847) 317-8153
Email: cbhd@cbhd.org

Information and ordering are also available through the Center's World Wide Web site on the Internet: *www.cbhd.org*.

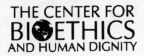

"BioEngagement"

*Making a Christian Difference
through Bioethics Today*

Edited by

NIGEL M. DE S. CAMERON,
SCOTT E. DANIELS,
and
BARBARA J. WHITE

WILLIAM B. EERDMANS PUBLISHING COMPANY
GRAND RAPIDS, MICHIGAN / CAMBRIDGE, U.K.

Published 2000 by Wm. B. Eerdmans Publishing Co.
255 Jefferson Ave. S.E., Grand Rapids, Michigan 49503 /
P.O. Box 163, Cambridge CB3 9PU U.K.

Printed in the United States of America

05 04 03 02 01 00   7 6 5 4 3 2 1

Library of Congress Cataloging-in-Publication Data

BioEngagement: making a Christian difference through bioethics today /
edited by Nigel M. de S. Cameron, Scott E. Daniels, and Barbara J. White,
p.   cm.   (Horizons in bioethics series)
ISBN 0-8028-4793-5 (pbk.: alk. paper)
1. Bioethics — Religious aspects — Christianity.
2. Medical ethics — Religious aspects — Christianity.
3. Christian ethics.   I. Cameron, Nigel M. de S.
II. Daniels, Scott E.   III.White, Barbara, 1940-   IV. Series.
QH332.B5173   2000
179′.1 — dc21

00-42693

www.eerdmans.com

Contents

CONTENTS

PART II
EDUCATION AND THE MEDIA

PART III
LAW AND PUBLIC POLICY

PART IV
HEALTH CARE

PART V
THE CHURCH

Contributors

Mary B. Adam, M.D., Clinical Lecturer, Department of Pediatrics, University of Arizona College of Medicine, Tucson, Ariz., U.S.A.

Francis J. Beckwith, Ph.D., Associate Professor of Philosophy, Culture, and Law, Trinity International University, California Campus, Santa Ana, Calif., U.S.A.

R. Geoffrey Brown, Ph.D., Senior Pastor and Head of Staff, Fletcher Hills Presbyterian Church, El Cajon, Calif., U.S.A.

Nigel M. de S. Cameron, Ph.D., Chairman, The Center for Bioethics and Human Dignity Advisory Board; Executive Chairman, The Centre for Bioethics and Public Policy, London, U.K.; Consultant, Strategic Futures, Bannockburn, Ill., U.S.A.

Samuel B. Casey, J.D., Executive Director, Christian Legal Society, Annandale, Va., U.S.A.

Scott E. Daniels, Ph.D., Former Deputy Secretary of Health and Human Resources for the Commonwealth of Virginia, Richmond, Va., U.S.A.

Marsha D. Fowler, Ph.D., Professor, Graduate Schools of Nursing and Theology, Azusa Pacific University, Azusa, Calif., U.S.A.

Teri N. Goudie, President, Goudie Media Services, Chicago, Ill., U.S.A.

Arnold G. Hyndman, Ph.D., Professor, Department of Cell Biology and

Neurobiology; Dean of Livingston College, Rutgers University, Piscataway, N.J., U.S.A.

John F. Kilner, Ph.D., Director, The Center for Bioethics and Human Dignity, Bannockburn, Ill., U.S.A.

Paul C. Madtes, Jr., Ph.D., Professor and Chair, Biology Department, Mount Vernon Nazarene College, Mount Vernon, Ohio, U.S.A.

Rt. Hon. Sir Brian Mawhinney, Ph.D., Member of Parliament, Privy Councillor, London, England, U.K.; former Minister of Health, U.K.

C. Ben Mitchell, Ph.D., Assistant Professor of Bioethics and Contemporary Culture, Trinity International University, Deerfield, Ill., U.S.A.

Dónal P. O'Mathúna, Ph.D., Professor of Bioethics and Chemistry, Mount Carmel College of Nursing, Columbus, Ohio, U.S.A.

Gregory W. Rutecki, M.D., Program Director, Internal Medicine Residency Program; Associate Professor of Medicine, Northwestern University Medical School, Evanston, Ill., U.S.A.

Terry A. Schlossberg, M.A., Executive Director, Presbyterians Pro-Life, Research, Education, and Care, Inc., Burke, Va., U.S.A.

David A. Sherwood, M.S.W., Ph.D., Professor of Social Work, Baylor University, Waco, Tex., U.S.A.

David L. Stevens, M.D., Executive Director, Christian Medical and Dental Society, Bristol, Tenn.; CBHD Advisory Board Member, Bannockburn, Ill., U.S.A.

Linda L. Treloar, R.N., Ph.D., Professor of Nursing, Scottsdale Community College; Practitioner, Educator, and Consultant, Scottsdale, Ariz., U.S.A.

Barbara J. White, R.N., Ed.D., Associate Professor, Department of Nursing, Regis University; Director, Congregational Health Partnerships, HealthONE Presbyterian/St. Luke's Medical Center, Denver, Colo., U.S.A.

Preface

In *Christ and Culture,* his classic essay on the predicament of Christianity and civilization, Richard Niebuhr outlines the kinds of relationship that different Christians at different times have engaged with the societies of their day. He foresees, rightly, that this question will matter a good deal to the church at the close of what have been called the "Christian centuries," and though it is now almost a half-century later (*Christ and Culture* first appeared in 1951 [reprinted New York: Harper and Row, 1975]), the onset of the third millennium leaves us with no better analysis than his. As it happens, the extraordinary persistence — indeed growth — of Christianity in North America during that earlier half-century, which could hardly have been predicted, has accentuated the problem.

For even as the church has held its own and expanded its appeal, the culture has moved in its seemingly inexorable drift into the post-Christian forms that have been emerging since the Enlightenment, the period of history that Christopher Dawson, in his fine book *The Crisis of Western Education* (1961; Steubenville, Ohio: Franciscan University Press, 1989), called "secularized Christendom." The contrast between our burgeoning churches and the scant impact that Christians have on public policy, or the arts, or the university, or the professions has been often noted. While some of the reasons are easier to identify than others (the determination with which so many evangelical Christians continue in their near-boycott of our public institutions is undoubtedly the most ironic of its causes), the challenge the situation presents could hardly be more pressing.

Nowhere is this development more evident than in bioethics. It is in bioethics, that point of intersection of the professions, the academy, and public policy, in which the dignity of the human being is constantly open to re-definition, and in which much of the best in our inheritance — medicine, science, the professional idea — is coming under withering fire from those whose values are radically distinct from the Judeo-Christian tradition. Our failure at the start of the new millennium to engage the culture in a degree which mirrors the size of our churches is distressing. Our failure in this realm of bioethics is particularly discouraging, since it is here that the assumptions of post-Christians are shaping their idea of what it is to be one of us.

Conversely, our opportunity to make a difference at this point is immense.

Western culture is still, even today, overshadowed by its Christian past and is desperately seeking moral leadership as it encounters the challenges posed by biotechnology. To suggest, however, that cultural engagement at this point is simply a rewarding option for Christians would be a mistake. Not only is it mandated by the doctrine of creation, in which God's human creatures are set in his world with a responsibility to act as his stewards over all he has made, but if the church fails to engage the culture for Christ, such neglect will compound the process already sadly visible around us, in which the distinctives of the Judeo-Christian worldview are incrementally lost as believers accommodate their moral vision to that of the world.

A glance at the contents page of this book illustrates the immense scope of our task, addressing as it does questions of public policy and law, education, media, and of course health care and the church itself. Niebuhr's *Christ and Culture* culminates in his model of the "transformation" of culture by Christ. Some chapters have been written by participants in the public arena, some by activists, some by academics and professionals. These writers are convinced that Christians are called to serve God in the myriad "secular" vocations of our day; that medicine and the other health-care professions, no less than the media, the university, and the three branches of government, participate in God's created *kosmos* and are therefore to be transformed for the gospel; that the fundamental mandate to be "in and not of" the world requires energetic engagement at every level as the dignity of human beings is at stake — the core issue in health care and the biosciences, as in every department of culture.

There are encouraging signs, including this book series and the associated Center for Bioethics and Human Dignity (CBHD). The Center lies at the heart of a network of physicians, nurses, academic bioethicists, Christian professional societies, and other groups who are united in their transformationist convictions and committed to the revival of Christian-Hippocratic ethics in the age of the Human Genome Project and its descendants. It is an international discussion, and the European institutions that partner with CBHD in sponsoring the journal *Ethics and Medicine* (the Centre for Bioethics and Public Policy in London, England, and the Lindeboom Instituut in Ede, The Netherlands) have also linked with CBHD in an international conference program in a series of European cities (including Bratislava, Budapest, and Brussels).

Many debts need to be paid as a volume of this kind is launched, and few can be listed here. We do wish to note our special thanks to our fellow authors whose timely and energetic work has been an example to us and has enabled this book to appear on schedule, and to The Center for Bioethics and Human Dignity, which has supported the production of this book, its director, Dr. John F. Kilner, and Miss Charity Bishop of its staff, who oversaw the collation of these papers.

Deerfield, Illinois Nigel M. de S. Cameron
January 14, 2000 Scott E. Daniels
Barbara J. White

PART I

CHRISTIAN VISION

Christian Leadership and Public Policy: Making a Difference

Rt. Hon. Sir Brian Mawhinney, MP, Ph.D.

We should start by defining what is this agent of difference that we have in mind. For me it is the fact and the application of the Christian faith in human relationships, both in the public arena and in our private experience. The word "Christian" has become a catchall in our modern society, frequently used simply as a claim to some element of "respectability." So let me say what I will mean when I use the word.

I will not be referring to ethical instructions or standards that people claim to have derived from the teaching of Jesus. Too often these amount to little more than a form of secular benchmarking. Nor will I be referring to the church networks and structures which cover this and other countries nor to the people who attend them, though Christians do go to church, for we are a worshiping people. I will not be laying claim, on behalf of those who appropriate the Christian name, to some form of moral superiority. Christians are not so defined because they are better or more worthy people than those around them, though Christians do seek to live their lives modeled on God's law. When I use the word "Christian," I will have in mind the Bible's teaching that Christians are those who have had their sins forgiven by God and, as a result, have entered into a personal relationship with the historic, incarnate, and living Jesus Christ.

God's forgiveness, available to us and through us to others, is the defining element of what it means to be a Christian, as the Lord's Prayer reminds us, "Forgive us, as we forgive others." There are many who will testify to the reality and the incalculable benefit of such a relationship with Jesus — both in their individual lives and in their public and professional experiences. We will also affirm that forgiveness of our sin, through trust in the risen Jesus, is the single most important thing in our lives.

I have been very fortunate. My earned Ph.D. afforded me recognition in the field of education, as I taught medical students in Iowa and London. As a Member of Parliament for over twenty years, I have experienced public recognition as I have had the privilege of representing hundreds of thousands of Cambridgeshire people in the House of Commons. I have been a Government Minister for over eleven years, and served for three years in the British Cabinet. My public service has been recognized nationally, both by being given a Knighthood and being made a Member of Her Majesty's Most Honorable Privy Council. Yes, I have been fortunate, but I also have that recognition in perspective. To me, political life is good and eternal life is better — and not just because the one is transitory and the other everlasting.

That personal relationship with Jesus can and does make a practical difference. Some months ago my wife and I received a letter from an American lady. She brought us up to date with her news and then told us of the exploits of her daughter at university. The pride in her choice of words was striking. She added that, without us and our introducing her to Jesus, there would have been no letter because there would have been no daughter. I reflected back to that evening, twenty years ago, when she rang our home. She had fled the United States and her parents, who were our close friends, for the anonymity of London — alone, pregnant, desperate, and with the promise of an abortion later that week. She came to the house and we fed her. A Christian doctor friend came over to answer her medical queries. She was agonizing about abortion. We talked about Jesus, his love for her, his forgiveness and strength, whatever she decided. She left us still undecided. We left her with God. We learned afterwards that she had given birth to a daughter. Twenty years later, we learned that that night she had also acquired a living faith. The forgiveness that Jesus offers does make a difference to individuals. We must affirm that as our first conclusion.

How that difference works itself out in the public arena will be a matter of contention between those who have a Christian faith and those who do not. It can be a matter of contention between Christians themselves. In the former case, the contention stems from our different presuppositions. After all, living and working in an eternal dimension ought to make us different from those who make decisions purely within a temporal framework. Knowing that human beings will someday be held accountable by God for what they have said, thought, and done — and omitted doing — should exert a different perspective on the values we espouse and the decisions we take.

And that perspective cannot be the same as one which stems from a belief that decisions have only an immediate and largely existential impact.

There is a world — an eternity — of difference between a credo based on "I want therefore I do" or "I do what I want" and one that is driven by the enquiry "What does Jesus expect of me?" The latter points to revealed truth and high standards of behavior, the former to whatever is the mood of the moment, what we can get away with, what would be nice or self-enhancing and what others of like inclination would do in similar circumstances. One takes, as its yardstick, God's divinely revealed moral absolutes; the other, the relative morality of the lowest common denominator in human behavior. If these two sets of presuppositions do not clash in the public arena, then we Christians are not effectively living our faith.

I have deliberately used language which tends to describe the opposite ends of a spectrum of moral reactions. Many would place themselves and their beliefs somewhere on that spectrum other than at its extremes. Indeed, the spectrum reflects the reality of our experience not least because our humanity, shaped in the image of God, retains within it instincts which are good, selfless, and which include a concern for others. However, the clash between absolutes and relativity is not thereby resolved.

Christians are different from others, because of forgiveness, and it is the networking of that difference which can make a difference more generally. Or, to use Jesus' words, Christians do, or should, bring an element of "salt" and "light" to contemporary affairs.

But there can also be contention between Christians. I regularly receive letters from voters in Britain on issues such as capital punishment, abortion, euthanasia, and homosexuality — all of them issues with a strong moral dimension and on which there has been much Christian teaching. They demand that I vote in a particular way because, they assert, that is clearly the Christian thing to do. My difficulty is that Christians write and require me to vote in diametrically different ways, even as they all tell me that theirs is the Christian way to make a difference. We need to explore behind that contradiction and seek both to understand what gives rise to it and how a more coherent and inclusive approach by Christians to such issues might be shaped.

We also need to grapple with the reality that Christians have, and will continue to have, different ideas on how matters of public policy should be resolved. At the same time we need to reflect upon in what circumstances it is both right and coherent for a single Christian voice to be heard. This is no idle musing. It is fundamental. I have Christian friends in all the main political parties in the United Kingdom. We pray, read the Bible, and have fellowship together. And, when the House of Commons' division bell rings we go our separate ways. Let us beware of suggesting, or even implying, that God goes with some of us or that he abandons others, whatever the issue. I have met and had fellowship with congressional Christians in Washington, D.C., whose party affiliations and different political approaches form no barrier, in either case, to the forgiveness of their sins; this despite the fact that they do lead to different policies in the public arena. Unless we can say that our God transcends Republican or Democratic Party ideas, we have no God.

I am privileged to be a trustee of Boston University. In this year's commencement address my attention focused on an intriguing reflection by our guest speaker, Dr. Henry Kissinger. He said, "When I started as a political advisor, politicians used to ask me what to think. Today, if they ask me anything, it is what to say." This is neither the time nor place to attempt to analyze the political legacies of either President Bill Clinton in the United States or Prime Minister Tony Blair in my country. They have transformed communication. The "soundbite" is here to stay, though I suspect long-term thinking will re-emerge. And Christians will want it to do so.

Many Christians will identify with what Dr. Kissinger said. We are engaged in a struggle, because of our beliefs, with those who, we suspect, think and operate more in step with this so-called modern thinking. Since the standards set by such thinking are all-embracing and, as a result, frequently less personally demanding, we Christians who are committed to biblical standards, are often found in a minority — which is never a position of strength in a democracy. Then, too often, we compound the problem. Instead of prioritizing our aims and objectives to achieve greater influence in the decision-making process, we retreat even more into the belief system which is important to us but irrelevant to so many others. In this way we ensure that we remain a powerless and frustrated minority. Instead, we should be seeking ways to move toward our goals by making common cause with others who want what we want — even if not for the same spiritually driven reasons.

In my experience, failure to address and resolve this fundamental dilemma contributes to the reality that we Christians, too often, make less of a public policy difference than we ought. If Christians are to be influential enough to make a difference in our society, then, based on my experience, there are two other issues we have to address.

First, we need to recognize that revealed law and politically driven legislation are not synonymous. Secondly, we have to affirm that there is a difference between what we Christians see as the "ends" of political activity and the "means" to achieve those ends. Let me look briefly at each of these in turn.

God revealed his nature and standards to us in order that we might appreciate and worship him and seek to please him by appropriating, as far as we can, his standards as our standards, by the power of his Spirit. When we fail to do that, we sin. His standards are simple to state even as they are hard to attain. Love the Lord your God with all your heart and your neighbor as yourself. Do not lie, lust, steal, or kill — and so on. In that sense they are about absolutes. Jesus did not go in much for mitigating circumstances, shades of gray, provocation, or other human rationalizations. He recognized, as the creed says, that we are all miserable sinners in need of divine forgiveness, and that forgiveness is his gracious gift.

It is, therefore, particularly inappropriate for Christians to believe, or even to advance the proposition that, in some meaningful, spiritual sense, God's law and man's law are somehow interchangeable. Of course we want to see legislation that is as compatible as possible with the Ten Commandments, but we do not believe that they are synonymous. Man's law sets parameters for acceptable — or to be more accurate, unacceptable — behavior. Such behavior is often, also, a breach of God's law. However, the human penalty is only temporal, not eternal. The corollary is also true. Keeping man's law is not the same as keeping God's law. It is possible never to be even arrested but still to go to hell.

When driving in Chicago, I have been reminded that American drivers take as relaxed a view of speed limits as do British drivers. In England I drive regularly from my home to my constituency, or district, as it would be called in America. The speed limit on the expressway is 70 mph. I seek to obey it while, on the outside lane, I am passed by cars, trucks, bicycles, and buggies! I shout at them to slow down — I and my colleagues passed a law that said 70 mph was to be the maximum — yet they go so fast they do not hear me! Our laws may constrain human behavior, but they cannot reach those parts of our being where change has to take place if people are to be fundamentally different. God's law can. I labor the point to emphasize it. Too often Christians press for a piece of legislation apparently buoyed by the hope that, if only it could be put on the statute book, certain aspects of our society of which we disapprove would be changed as a consequence. Even if we passed laws to prohibit murder, tax evasion, drug trafficking, homosexual acts, abortion, child abuse, or whatever is your particular "bête noir" — and in all cases we have — the practices would continue.

Human sin is not amenable to cleansing by Act of Congress or Parliament. We Christians know and believe that, even if sometimes, by our words and actions, we deny it. This, of course, is not a reason for washing our hands of the legislative process on the grounds that it is irrelevant. It is not irrelevant, and we *should* try to influence it. However, recognizing that it is never the transforming power of God, offers us the opportunity to make common cause with others who share our assessment of what is in the common good but who do not necessarily share our Christian presuppositions. Third World debt might be a case in point.

The second issue relates to what we believe public policy should reflect and how best to achieve this. In both the U.S. and the U.K. we are privileged that the "ends" of our political processes are largely a matter of shared political agreement. We want our countries to be strong, secure and free from external or internal threat; we want our people to enjoy the provision of good social services, including education and health, in a form that benefits all, with no one excluded for financial reasons. We want them to be protective of the rights and dignities of all, and to prosper and provide employment which satisfies those who want to work, or have to. We want governments that encourage opportunity and respect individual privacy. And so on. These "ends" have largely been shaped by our shared Judeo-Christian heritage and beliefs. In both our countries — perhaps more in the U.K. than in the U.S. — we generate the political heat by debating the "means" to achieve these politically agreed "ends" not the "ends" themselves.

Let me illustrate the point I intend to convey. Christians affirm the fundamental right of government to raise and spend taxes. That was one of the imperatives of Paul's message in his letter to the Roman Christians (chapter 13). It was also Jesus' message when he told his disciples to render unto Caesar the things that are Caesar's (Matthew 22) and by his identifying with tax collectors. Paying tax is as much an imperative of our faith as is telling the truth or thinking purely. Incidentally, I am sorry if that means you have to revise your view of the taxman and that binding date in April! What the Bible does not do, however, is give any indication about what tax rates should apply; how much tax should be raised, or whether direct or indirect taxation is preferable. Those "means" to achieve an agreed, divine "end" are for politicians and the public to decide.

In deciding how Christians can make a difference in public policy terms, it is important to differentiate clearly between these two truths. "Ends" are what we are committed to, arising from our faith. "Means" are how we decide to try to achieve them — with the caveat, of course, that they are moral, legal, and, to us Christians, not incompatible with the nature of our God. It is this distinction that makes it possible for Christians to be members of all political parties, and none. This truth also provides the basis for rejecting the contention of those who claim that Christians cannot become involved in politics, because to do so requires them to compromise.

Politics does involve compromise. Every piece of congressional or state legislation is a compromise — or gives effect to a consensus, if you prefer this more delicate expression. The end products — Acts of Congress — seldom, if ever, reflect exactly what the sponsors initially intended. To achieve the support necessary for law-making, changes had to be agreed in exchange for votes. Incidentally, that does not mean that the legislative end product is necessarily worse than the originally envisaged bill. It just means that it is different. My business is seldom about 100 percent and 0 percent of an issue or decision — it is usually about trying to achieve 53 percent or 66 percent or avoiding 45 percent or 29 percent. As Edmund Burke said, "all government, indeed every human benefit and enjoyment, every virtue and every prudent act, is founded on compromise and barter." Before you rush to condemn what we do on your behalf, please pause for just for a moment.

I have served on the medical faculties of two universities. When we came together to decide what to teach our students, many suggestions were made. Eventually we had to choose and decide, else nothing would ever have been taught. In that process almost everyone had to give up some cherished ambition or agree to some aspect of the syllabus that he or she thought inappropriate or unnecessary. We all compromised in order to make progress. I have served on church governing bodies in three denominations on two continents. Those who served with me were spiritual people, wanting the best for their "flock." Yet our views of what was "best" frequently diverged widely. Some held to their views with tenacity. Others compromised more easily. But the agreed program, which emerged after argument, discussion, and prayer, did constitute a compromise for those present. My wife Betty and I have been married for thirty-four years. We often find that, when together, we want to do different things. She wants to do one thing. I want to do another. So we compromise. We do what she wants! (Well, nearly always.)

It is in the nature of human relationships that when two or more people come together, they discover that their views and ambitions are different — sometimes by a little, sometimes by a lot. If action is required, if decisions are needed, then compromise is necessary. As John Donne reminded us, "no man is an island." Yet this inevitability of compromise remains especially difficult for conservative and evangelical Christians who have been raised on God's absolutes, with the added certainty that those who disagreed with us were just plain wrong. In truth we have had too little coherent Bible teaching on the nature of compromise and on the fundamental importance of it being acceptable to compromise in pursuit of the "means" of politics, while it is never defensible to compromise the pillars of our faith from which flow our political "ends." If we are to make a difference in the market place, then much more attention needs to be paid to this area of our witness, with teaching to follow.

Let me touch on one other distraction and source of damage to public

Christian witness. Again, I start with an example. Every Good Friday morning, Betty and I join other Christians from local churches in Peterborough in a Walk of Witness through the streets of that city — which I represent. The march concludes with an open-air service in Cathedral Square. One year, during the 1980s, while waiting for the service to begin, I found myself standing immediately behind two ladies, one of whom recognized me. Although I was only a few feet from her, she proceeded to talk to her friend in a loud stage whisper, clearly intending that I should hear. "I see the Member of Parliament is here," she said. "He claims to be a Christian, you know. I don't see how he can be, he doesn't support the Campaign for Nuclear Disarmament." For those who are not familiar with the name, CND was the umbrella organization in the United Kingdom for all those who, during the period of heightened tension with the communist world, wanted the West to initiate unilateral nuclear disarmament. Now, a moral case could be made for such a political stance. Many Christians made it and believed it. More believed that a morally stronger case could be made for deterring would-be aggressors by stressing the cost to them of launching their nuclear warheads in our direction. With a doctorate in radiation biology, I know better than most the awfulness of the consequences of nuclear attack, and I judged deterrence better than one-sided disarmament. That, too, was the policy of both our governments, and it prevailed.

My point is not to argue the merits of the two approaches. Both could be construed as moral. Both had Christian adherents and advocates. Individual Christians had to choose. My point is that this dear Christian lady added support for CND to the good news of Jesus Christ as an essential extra prerequisite to saving faith — a further "hoop" through which I was expected to pass before she could consider my Christian faith genuine. No such prerequisite "hoop" exists in the Bible, or church teaching. Yet, frequently, Christians adopt the same approach toward other Christians. Too often we are tempted to judge people's faith by whether or not they conform to or can "pass" the extra requirements *we* impose on them; to put it bluntly, whether or not they agree with us.

Two consequences follow. Christian is divided from Christian, and the "salt" and "light," which Jesus said we were to be in society, is diluted. We need to differentiate carefully between revelation and manifesto.

Let me turn briefly to two issues which lie at the heart of our considerations in this book, namely the protection of life and what constitutes human dignity. Recently, I came across some contemporary United States statistics. They are examples of the risks estimated to increase the annual chance of death by one in one million: smoking 1.4 cigarettes, spending one hour in a coal mine, living two days in New York or Boston, traveling ten miles by bicycle, flying a thousand miles by jet, one clear x-ray in a good hospital, eating forty pounds of peanut butter, drinking thirty 12-oz. cans of diet soda, and living 150 years within twenty miles of a nuclear power plant.

In the U.S., many thousands die each year as a result of the use of guns, both legally and illegally held. Thousands of others are killed on the roads — through speeding and the effect of alcohol and drugs. Yet, overwhelmingly, when life and death issues are considered as matters of public policy, the Christian voice is raised most loudly or sometimes heard only on the issue of abortion. Do Christians have no views, for example, about issues arising from children bringing guns into schools and, if so, how effectively do we pursue them? Do not misunderstand me. Christian voices should be raised about abortion. The death toll of unborn children is enormous and indefensible. Abortion has become, to so many, little more than a convenient alternative method of birth control. Sanctity of life issues have been sidelined in the operating theatre. I am not a supporter of abortion. Over the years that has been the basis of my voting record. Like many of you, one of the beliefs that defines me, my faith, and its practice is that human beings were made in the image of God.

Much that is important and practical flows from that truth, including a prohibition on lightly taking life for reasons of convenience, or indeed inconvenience. This chapter is not an essay on abortion but comments on being a Christian in the public arena. Within that constraint, and drawing on my own experience, I want to make three simple points.

First, it is important that the Christian voice continues to be heard in defense of the defenseless. Jesus spoke for those who were weak and disadvantaged and who had no advocates. So should we. Our "salty" influence can help retard the effect of that element of rottenness in our society that stems from the fact that men and women insist on acting without regard to God's law. It may even reduce the unwarranted taking of life.

My second point is a less comfortable one. Some Christians go further than simply opposing abortion and rejecting any arguments in favor of mitigating circumstances. They make this issue *the* defining spiritual issue as they converse, work, worship, and have fellowship with other Christians. To them it becomes a similar extra "hoop" to the one imposed by my Peterborough constituent. They may recognize that others have been "born again" and have had their sins forgiven; but if they are not "sound" on abortion then they can hardly be thought to be Christian. It may be that every Christian generation has an issue on which it feels compelled to speak out. It is right to do so. But it is equally right that we should not confuse either others or ourselves about what constitute the essentials of our faith. If our fundamental belief is the sanctity of life, why are we heard less compellingly on all those other life-threatening issues I have mentioned? I know from experience in both our countries that, although I have taken the precaution of pre-stating my own view on abortion, the very fact of my saying what I have said may cause some to doubt the sincerity and even question the genuineness of my faith. That should worry all of us. My point here is not an abortion point; it is "an effective Christian witness in the public arena" point.

In both Britain and the United States we Christians are in a minority. Our presuppositions are not the majority ones, despite our affirmation that it is In God We Trust. The moral relativism of our age has enticed many of our neighbors and elected representatives away from Christianity. They will not be persuaded to our viewpoint simply by our proclaiming that we have the mind of God on a subject. To make a difference in the public arena, we will need to develop arguments that will seem more compelling and relevant to those who do not share our Christian presuppositions, than do our present arguments and assertions. And we will have to form alliances with those who share our goals, for whatever democratic reason, if we are to have any chance of changing contemporary mores.

In the U.K. and maybe in the U.S., legislation and practice will not change unless and until the bigger battle over standards, values, and beliefs has been won. At the moment too many Christians are not engaged. They continue to exercise their faith within the confines of their churches and Christian fellowships. That is fine and rewarding, but it militates against change in the wider society. And too many Christians are so consumed with the rightness of their cause that they seldom wonder why it remains a losing one.

When Christians are tempted to reject the real Christian faith of those who may disagree with them on any moral issue, the effect is counter productive in the public arena, however "satisfying" it may be to individuals. Divisiveness within the body of Christ makes the job of Christians, like me, in that public arena, more difficult, for it gives non-believers a rationale to reject our message. If the issue is "making a difference" in public policy, then we need to ask ourselves, in both countries, what difference have our tactics made, thus far? And is the cause of Christ assisted, if any issue close to the heart of faithful Christians becomes identified, fairly or not, with a particular political party's policy?

I said I wanted to make three points about the sanctity of life from the vantage point of the public arena. Non-Christians regularly ask me why, when it comes to sanctity of life issues, they hear so much about abortion and so little about so much else that is indefensible from a Christian perspective.

Do we not care about these other issues? Or do we suffer from tunnel-vision faith? Abortion is *so* important, I hear many say. I agree. But so are other issues. The very imbalance in our approach may cause some, without our presuppositions, to question the reality of our commitment to life from God and people created in the image of God. Even worse, they may question whether God loves some more, because of their experiences, than he loves others? These observations should cause us to reflect on whether, if we were less selective in our crusades, we would become more compelling in the public arena, as people saw the uniform breadth of our concern for inter-related life issues.

Let me turn now to human dignity. For many in the public arena, this phrase already carries different connotations from those associated with some Christian uses of the phrase. I think of it as describing and reinforcing the special nature of mankind's creation by God: made in his image. In the public arena, however, it is more likely to mean affirming whatever choice people make about themselves and their relationships. To deny people their own free choice is, we are told, to deny them their dignity. However, this approach requires more analytical assessment. "Free choice" has become the slogan, almost the market brand, of our age. It carries with it the implication that, by definition, the "choices" people make are always good ones because we have decided that choice is good per se. Although we understand that having the opportunity to choose is different from the choices that are made, and that the former can be good while the latter may be bad, the public analysis is seldom even this rigorous.

Secondly, the word "free" also implies to many that any choice made must be a good one. The assumption in this case is that we would only choose the best for ourselves when unconstrained by any external pressures. After all, we all know what is best for ourselves, don't we? Well, no, actually, we do not, if the evidence is anything to go by. One marriage in three in the U.K. ends in divorce and the proportion is rising. The percentage of relationships outside marriage that do not last is even higher. Choosing lifestyles that end in helpless drug addiction or in prison hardly commend themselves as good choices — free or otherwise. Neither does becoming a mother or father at fifteen. Christians cannot endorse systems, even popular ones, that are value free or, even more importantly, belief free. To do so is to deny what we believe about people's need for God in their lives and the importance of acknowledging their dependence on him.

We believe that "human dignity" is found in "the image of God" and that sets us at odds with the majority in the public arena. So, again, we find ourselves having to contend with the majority — and slowly losing the battle.

Let me illustrate what I mean. In Britain, if actuarial projections prove correct, those who are married will be in a minority relationship by the year 2010. In the U.S., the election of a bishop who believes in same gender "weddings" appears likely before too long. And the battle to equate heterosexual and homosexual relationships in the eyes of society, the law, and the church, has already largely slipped beyond the control — and maybe even the influence — of those who believe that God does not equate such practices. If God does make the difference, how is it that so many Christians in the public arena appear willing to side with the contemporary definition of human dignity rather than the revealed one? Should Paul's warning to the Romans, not to let the world squeeze us into its mould, be ringing in our ears? Where are the Christian exegetical and pastoral support systems which those Christians who do take a stand in the public arena need, when faced with considerable pressure and, at least in elected politics, even abuse? Without such systems, making a difference publicly remains more difficult than it should be.

Finally, I want to bring into sharper focus two threads which have been running through much of what I have been saying. The first is that those of us who are Christians should more carefully differentiate between what it is we hold in trust for God — those things which we believe cannot be the object of compromise — and what are the human and relational means we can use, change, and adapt to help us fulfil our spiritual objectives. Ambiguity and confusion between these reduce our chances to make a difference.

The second thread has been more implicit. We find ourselves in a marketplace of ideas and spiritual remedies; we are literally engaged in a battle for people's souls. Yet, frequently, we pay little more than lip service to the importance of communicating the good news of Jesus Christ, in the sort of principled and persuasive way that will catch and hold people's attention in the public arena.

During my lifetime, I have been told that the two greatest threats to my physical and spiritual well-being were communism and materialism. The one was godless; the other the elevation of the pursuit and love of money as a substitute God. Personally, I believe an equally potent third threat has emerged. It is a cynicism that values nothing and believes everything, and therefore nothing. It is found in the classroom, the hospital ward, the law court, the church, government, and, perhaps preeminently, in the media. These are the areas covered by this book, so the issue lies at the heart of our deliberations. Cynicism, in its most insidious form, surfaces again and again in the media. I say "most insidious," in part, because it is through the media and the Internet that we are so regularly exposed to valueless messages. Belief systems are of little effect if they do not work hand in hand with the means of challenging, combating, and converting those who believe in other gods, or in none. If we are to be heard and taken seriously, we need to be distinguished by solid defensible beliefs and persuasive presentation. Anyone operating in the public arena will tell you that.

As a Christian Member of Parliament my reputation is largely defined by the media. How they project me is how I am "seen" by millions of people who have no other way of "knowing" me. Media presuppositions — and the way they are given expression — are therefore intimately linked with the way the Christian message is received and perceived more widely. Let me give you a very simple illustration. In the early 1980s my party decided to organize a day conference in London on "Conservatism and Christianity." The then Bishop of London, the Rt. Rev. Graham Leonard, was invited to give the morning keynote address, and I was invited to chair that first session. About two hundred people were present, and there was much media interest. Eventually, after the audience quietened and the cameras were rolling, I said, "Our God is not a Conservative, a Socialist, Liberal or Social Democrat. He is God. And that is where we start our conference." As I drove to the House of Commons, I heard the newsreader on the BBC's lunchtime bulletin tell millions of listeners that a Conservative MP had *admitted* (my emphasis) this morning that God was *not* a Conservative. Just that — no more explanation. That was the only message conveyed. This incident tells you more about the BBC than it does about me, about God, or about the conference. If we are to make a difference in the public arena, we cannot afford to ignore the means of communication. That has been my repeated experience.

The detailed discussion, models, and strategies are still to come. But it is right to remind ourselves, at the beginning of this volume, of the incalculable benefits we enjoy as children of God engaged in spiritual warfare; for we will never make a difference if we are daunted by the task at hand. First, we are loved — irrespective of how we cope with the pressures of the public arena. A wise and godly Christian once gave me advice which, in my life, has been almost defining. "Remember, Brian," he said, "there is nothing you can do or achieve that will make God love you more, and there is nothing you can do, no matter how bad, that will make God love you less. And he has already shown the extent and depth of his love for you when he gave his Son to die for you." Secondly, not only are we loved, we are also powerful, for through God's Spirit we have available to us God's power that "upholds all things," that "made the blind see" and the "lame walk," that "raised Jesus himself from the dead" and "defeated the devil." Now that is what I call "power." And, as Elijah discovered, spiritually those who are for us are more than those who are against us. Thirdly, as we are loved and powerful so we are forgiven. That is the fulcrum around which the gospel of Jesus, lived out in the words and lives of his people, can change lives. As the modern hymn puts it,

"God forgave my sin in Jesus' name,
I've been born again in Jesus' name,
And in Jesus' name I come to you,
To share His love as He told me to."

"He said, freely, freely you have received
Freely, freely give,
Go in my name and because you believe
Others will know that I live."

And, finally, we are called — to be faithful only to our heavenly calling. To the relief of many, we are not called to be successful — just to be faithful. To be "salt" in a rotting world and "light" in a dark one. To be faithful to what we have learned and experienced and to the need to explain and affirm the One in whom we have placed our trust. To be reflectors of the grace and truth of Jesus to the world he made and loves. That is all. And while each of us has been given a manifestation of the Spirit for the common good — it is the job of God's Spirit to determine the increase. Throughout the pages of this book, authors will examine how we can put these divine blessings to use in order to maximize the difference Christians can make in the various public arenas to which we have been called. It is an exciting prospect.

A Biblical Mandate
for Cultural Engagement

John F. Kilner, Ph.D.

Does it make a difference in this world to be a Christian? Or, to put it differently, can a Christian make a difference in this world? The answer to both questions is "Yes, but. . . ."

It makes a difference to be a Christian, in the sense that "Christ-ians" — people in whom the Spirit of Jesus Christ dwells — can be profoundly different than they would be without Christ. And yet, all too often those of us who intend to be different are not. Our values or our relationships, for example, are sometimes so thoroughly shaped by the fallen world that they are indistinguishable from those of people who hold to the world's values. Similarly, Christians can indeed make a tremendous difference in this world. In fact, history and the present day are filled with powerful examples of those who have. And yet, all too often we do not have such an impact; or if we have any impact at all, it involves such compromise that God is little glorified.

How have we fallen into this state? Simply put, in our desire to reach the world we have become too much like the world. We have underestimated the dangers of becoming like the world, and we have become willing to do anything — to be anything — in order to make a difference. Of course, we won't *literally* do or be anything, for there are certain things so obviously un-Christian that none of us can deceive ourselves into engaging in them. And yet, the influence of the world is so strong, and we are at times so unwary, that it is amazing how adept we become at rationalizing why we should be able to act in a particular worldly way.

The problem here is that in our well-intentioned commitment to the

17

world that God has made we have paid insufficient attention to the Word that God has given. In sending his people out to make a difference, God has always armed them with his spoken, incarnate, or written Word. We have the privilege today to have God's written Word, the Bible, to clarify and interpret the guidance God has given us throughout the ages. It is this Word that gives us a vantage point from which to see a true way to make a constructive impact around us — a perspective from which to distinguish this way from the attractive but counterproductive approaches the world has to offer.

How can we best discover what the Bible would teach us about making a difference in the world? In the space available, it is at least possible to sketch a framework for our understanding by examining various places in the New Testament where the word kosmos appears, since kosmos is the word most often used in the New Testament for the "world" and "culture" we are eager to engage. (John alone uses it more than a hundred times.) In fact, we can even use kosmos instead of its English counterparts in our discussion of the Bible's teaching, in order to remind us that we are not interested here so much in the way people commonly use the words "culture" and "world" as we are in the way the Bible uses them.

Needless to say, there are many ways that the biblical material could be organized. For instance, kosmos sometimes refers to the world that God has created: in a morally good sense that looks back to the creation, in a neutral sense as simply the setting in which people live today, or in a way that looks ahead to God's future intentions for the world (though "kingdom" language is more often used in this last context). More often, however, kosmos refers negatively to the present world that has wandered far from God and God's ways. While organizing this chapter by such categories would be one viable way to proceed, the interplay of these categories as they appear in the biblical texts would be partly lost in the process. So an alternative approach will be followed here — though every attempt will be made to indicate which of the above contexts is relevant in each reference to kosmos.

As we explore the New Testament writings, we will find *challenges, tasks, obstacles,* and *resources* for our engagement with the kosmos. Knowing and handling these appropriately will go a long way toward enabling us to truly make a God-honoring, constructive difference in today's world. Rather than simply lumping together the entire set of New Testament materials, we will listen to the harmonious but distinct voices of four smaller sets of New Testament writings: the Synoptic Gospels (Matthew, Mark, and Luke),[1] the writ-

---

1. The Book of Acts is also included here since it was written by one of the Synoptic Gospel authors, Luke.

ings of John,[2] the letters of Paul,[3] and, when they add new thoughts not found elsewhere, the other New Testament letters.[4] These four sets of writings not only reinforce one another, but help us to see the same reality from different vantage points.

Challenges

Synoptic Gospels

If we are to engage the kosmos effectively, we first need to appreciate the challenges before us. In the Synoptic Gospels we learn that the kosmos is a fallen place in which sin is unavoidable. "Woe to the kosmos because of the things that cause people to sin! Such things must come, but woe to the one through whom they come!"[5] While evil deeds are done by individuals, who are responsible for that evil, there is a sense here in which Jesus views the kosmos as a corporate entity about which he speaks this "woe" — much the same as he speaks woes against the rich Pharisees and other evildoers. The kosmos is not just a setting in which individuals may sin; it is a setting that is itself necessarily sinful. In fact, the synoptic authors often casually refer to the kosmos as the fallen creation, a place marked by hiddenness, suffering, and death.[6]

The kosmos — with its values, people, and structures that exist without reference to God — stands in stark contrast to the kingdom of God, which encompasses values, people, and structures dedicated to God. For example, in the words of Jesus: "Do not set your heart on what you will eat or drink; do

2. Included here are all of the writings claiming to be written by John (John; 1, 2, and 3 John; Revelation), since they were all either written by John or intentionally written to resemble John's perspective more than the perspective of other authors. Issues of authorship need not be debated here since the purpose of this essay is not to distinguish one New Testament author's outlook from another. Rather, it is to describe the full teaching of the New Testament regarding Christian engagement with the kosmos.

3. Included here are all of the writings claiming to be written by Paul (Romans, 1 and 2 Corinthians, Galatians, Ephesians, Philippians, Colossians, 1 and 2 Thessalonians, 1 and 2 Timothy, Titus, Philemon), since they were all either written by Paul or intentionally written to resemble Paul's perspective more than the perspective of other authors. See note 2 regarding authorship issues.

4. Included here are Hebrews, James, 1 and 2 Peter, and Jude.

5. Matt. 18:7. (All Bible quotations in this chapter are based on the New International Version.)

6. Matt. 13:35; 24:21; Luke 11:50.

not worry about it. For the pagan kosmos runs after all such things, and your Father knows that you need them. But seek his kingdom, and these things will be given to you as well. Do not be afraid, little flock. . . . Sell your possessions and give to the poor."[7] Whereas the kosmos focuses on goods, the kingdom focuses on God — running after goods versus resting in God. The kosmos is characterized by fear, the kingdom by faith; the kosmos by grasping, the kingdom by giving. Recognizing the striking differences between the kosmos and the kingdom is an important first step in preparing to engage the kosmos in a way that remains true to the kingdom.

Writings of John

The apostle John also writes of the "viewpoint of the kosmos,"[8] emphasizing that it is very different from the outlook of God and God's kingdom: "Everything in the kosmos — the cravings of sinful people, the lust of their eyes and the boasting of what they have and do — comes not from the Father but from the kosmos."[9] Elsewhere John expands on how different the kosmos is from the trinitarian God. It is an arena in which the Father's presence,[10] the Holy Spirit's truth,[11] and Jesus Christ's peace are absent.[12] For example, according to Jesus himself, "In me you may have peace. In this kosmos you will have trouble." Why? Because Christians will follow in the footsteps of the One for whom they are named — the One who observed that "The kosmos . . . hates me because I testify that what it does is evil."[13] Indeed, the kosmos and the kingdom are two very different realms, with very different standards. Jesus insists: "My kingdom is not of this kosmos . . . my kingdom is from another place."[14]

John not only fleshes out the kosmos-kingdom contrast in greater detail, but he adds the observation that the kosmos is subject to demonic rule. It is filled with many deceivers and false prophets who are empowered by the spirit of the antichrist.[15] In fact, "the whole kosmos is under the control of

7. Luke 12:29-33a.
8. 1 John 4:5.
9. 1 John 2:16.
10. John 13:1; 16:28.
11. John 14:17; 1 John 4:5-6.
12. John 16:33; 14:27.
13. John 7:7.
14. John 18:36.
15. 1 John 4:1, 3; 2 John 7.

the evil one,"[16] he writes, echoing Jesus' own description of Satan as "the prince of this kosmos."[17]

Letters of Paul

Like John's writings, Paul's letters affirm many of the insights about the kosmos presented in other New Testament writings. The letter to the Ephesians in particular underscores John's insight that if we are to engage the kosmos, we must be prepared to wrestle with demonic forces: "Our struggle is not against flesh and blood, but against the rulers, against the authorities, against the powers of this dark kosmos and against the spiritual forces of evil in the heavenly realms."[18] By clarifying that there are demonic beings at work specifically in our world, this passage warns us not to approach engaging the kosmos as if it were simply a secular challenge to be tackled with our human mental and physical abilities alone.

One problem with such a human approach, as Paul sees it, is that it is "worldly." It uses the same faulty human wisdom to get us out of our current predicament as that which got us into it in the first place. But, "The wisdom of this kosmos is foolishness in God's sight."[19] According to the letters to the Colossians and Galatians, such wisdom operates on "principles" and "rules" that have an appearance of wisdom, but are without basis.[20] In the realm of bioethics we are all too familiar with such principles. The kosmos is under bondage to such principles as autonomy and utility. These empty principles have an almost religious attraction, as if they will lead us to personal and social happiness. However, by failing to acknowledge God or to recognize people as created in the image of God, they perpetuate and augment the inner emptiness and oppression of the weak that ravage the kosmos.

Other Letters

The other letters of the New Testament see the separation between the kosmos and God as so great that James warns: "Don't you know that friendship with the kosmos is hatred toward God? Anyone who chooses to be a

---

16. 1 John 5:19.
17. John 12:31.
18. Eph. 6:12; cf. 2:2.
19. 1 Cor. 3:19; cf. 1:20-21.
20. Col. 2:20-23; Gal. 4:3.

friend of the kosmos becomes an enemy of God."[21] This strong language becomes more understandable when we recall that there is active demonic involvement in the kosmos. As Peter reminds us, "Your enemy the devil prowls around like a roaring lion looking for someone to devour. . . . Your brothers and sisters throughout the kosmos are undergoing the same kind of sufferings."[22]

Tasks

Synoptic Gospels

In the face of such formidable challenges, what are our God-given tasks? How are Christians to make a difference in the kosmos? The heart of the matter for the authors of the Synoptic Gospels involves putting faithfulness to God above achieving worldly success. Luke reminds us, quoting Paul, that "The God who made the kosmos and everything in it is the Lord. . . . And he is not served by human hands, as if he needed anything, because he himself gives all people life and breath and everything else."[23] Despite its current rebellion and fallen state, the kosmos was created by God and is loved by God; God knows better than anyone else how to constructively engage it. As Lord over everything, God could fix every bioethical problem in an instant. We would do well to tackle such issues in the ways God directs, rather than developing our own human strategies — perhaps following worldly techniques — in a vain attempt to improve on God's abilities or timing. It does not matter where in the lifespan a bioethical issue arises — whether in the womb ("life"), near birth ("breath"), or later ("everything else"). God's way is the best way, and it is our task to learn as much about it as we can.

Nevertheless, there is a balance to maintain. Our task is not to sit idly by and trust God to do all that needs doing. On the one hand, if you are a believer who is willing to do anything to help God's kingdom supplant the kosmos, you must rest in what God has already done: "The kingdom [has been] prepared for you since the creation of the kosmos. . . ."[24] On the other hand, to participate in that kingdom you must faithfully demonstrate the heart of God to an errant world by loving God enough to live out God's pri-

---

21. James 4:4.
22. 1 Peter 5:8-9; cf. James 4:4-7.
23. Acts 17:24-25.
24. Matt. 25:34.

orities — even if they are not valued by the world. If you do not act on such priorities as caring for the poor and weak, especially among God's people, then the Lord says: "'Whatever you did not do for one of the least of these, you did not do for me.' Then they will go away to eternal punishment, but the righteous to eternal life."[25]

Writings of John

To this theme of faithfulness John adds a fuller account of the Christian's tasks in the world. Chapter 17 of his Gospel is especially significant in this regard, since he explicitly looks ahead to future generations — even to us. He indicates, in effect, that of all the things Jesus has talked about, one thing that will be especially applicable and important to those to come will be what he has taught about how to relate to the kosmos. Accordingly, after praying for his disciples, Jesus continues: "My prayer is not for them alone. I pray also for those who will believe in me through their message." Consider these verses from Jesus' prayer to the Father for those who follow him: "They are still in the kosmos. . . . My prayer is not that you take them out of the kosmos. . . . They are not of the kosmos even as I am not of it. . . . As you sent me into the kosmos, I have sent them into the kosmos."[26]

First, we are to resist the tendency to respond to the fallenness of the kosmos by withdrawing from it (v. 15); instead we are to remain "in" it (v. 11) in order to make a difference. Yet, more precisely, we are not to be merely "in" the kosmos, we are to be "into" it — not just present but proactive, strategically engaged in impacting it. Yet Jesus cautions that we must be careful in the process not to become "of" the kosmos. We are to be engaged but not entangled. Otherwise, rather than shaping the world we will instead be shaped by it. An apt summary of Jesus' teaching recorded here and elsewhere[27] by John is not the familiar expression that we should be "in the world but not of it." Rather, it is that we should be "*into* the world, not of it!" We must make sure that we are "in the world, not out of it." But that is just our position, not our mission. Once we are in position, then we must proactively engage.

What should this engagement look like? John has much to say about that as well. First, in line with the Synoptic Gospels, engagement must remain

25. Matt. 25:45-46 (cf. vv. 35, 40).
26. John 17:11, 15-16, 18.
27. On not being "of" the kosmos, see also John 8:23; on being "in" the kosmos, see also John 13:1; on being "into" the kosmos, see also 1 John 4:9 (cf. John 11:27).

faithful to God. As important as it is to make a difference by engaging the kosmos, it is more important to remain true to God in the process, for "The kosmos and its desires pass away, but the one who does the will of God lives forever."[28] A faithful engagement must necessarily be a redemptive engagement, not a judgmental one. Although it is so much easier as we engage bioethical issues to focus on critiquing and discrediting the "other side," a fully Christian engagement must endeavor to heal and restore, not merely to condemn. In this we are to follow Christ's example.

It is easy to be misled at this point, as many have been, by misunderstanding Christ as primarily a righteous judge. Jesus did indeed say "For judgment I have come into this world. . . ."[29] Yet several chapters later in the Gospel of John he is quoted as saying "I did not come to judge the world."[30] How can these both be true? The key is in specifying who is doing the judging. It is God the Father, not Jesus Christ redemptively at work engaging the kosmos. After saying "I did not come to judge the world," Jesus goes on to clarify: "but [I came] to save it."[31] Christ's mission — and ours as we follow him — is to restore those who have abandoned God's life-affirming ways. Jesus Christ is the "light of the kosmos" who brings sight to the blind and exposes the blindness of those who mistakenly think they can see.[32] As we, with him, seek to bring healing light to the kosmos — and people separate into those willing to change and those who are not — God the Father takes responsibility for the judgment that must result. Accordingly, immediately after saying he did not come to judge the world but to save it, Jesus adds that "There is a judge for the one who rejects me and does not accept my words . . . : the Father." Even God the Father does not welcome the opportunity to judge, but does everything possible, out of love, to avoid punishing people: "God so loved the kosmos that he gave his one and only Son, that whoever believes in him shall not perish but have eternal life. For God did not send his Son into the kosmos to condemn the kosmos but to save the kosmos through him."[33] Neither should we condemn the kosmos or those in it.

In addition to our engagement with the kosmos being faithful and redemptive, it is also to be restorative. Our engagement is to be not merely one of ideas and ethical positions, but also one of meeting specific needs. People recognized Jesus as "the Prophet who is to come into the kosmos," notes John,

28. 1 John 2:17.
29. John 9:39.
30. John 12:47.
31. See also John 3:17.
32. John 9:5, 39; cf. 8:26.
33. John 3:16-17.

when he joined meeting their physical hunger with his teaching ministry.[34] So today the transforming love of Christ is unleashed not simply by telling people that abortion or assisted suicide are wrong, but rather by combining such statements with action initiatives designed to meet the social, economic, physical, emotional, and spiritual needs that incline people to such practices in the first place.

Jesus additionally provides a model for us in the way that he engages the kosmos publicly and urgently. He intentionally speaks "openly to the kosmos" rather than hiding from the kosmos what he is truly about.[35] Furthermore, he brings a sense of urgency to the task in conjunction with his claim to be the "light of the kosmos." Lest we miss that he is not talking here merely about his own work in the world but about our tasks as well, he inserts a "we" where we would normally expect an "I": "As long as it is day, we must do the work of him who sent me. Night is coming, when no one can work."[36] We must not take for granted the opportunity *we* have right now to engage the kosmos. We may only have another year or two to make a difference — or less.

Letters of Paul

Paul, meanwhile, helps us to wrestle with the fact that ethics is unavoidably related to what is true. For example, if a person is precious — whether because created in the image of God or otherwise — then ethics requires us to respect and protect that person. If a person has no greater significance than that of a rock, then no special protection is normally required.

The difficulty Christians encounter in the kosmos is that their understanding of what is true about the world is different from that of others. Whereas many consider autonomy ethics (or an ethics of choice) to be manifestly true since they see no higher ethical authority than the individual, Christians must respond, with Paul, that "You are not your own; you were bought at a price."[37] Similarly, many find that a utilitarian pursuit of the greatest good for the greatest number, whatever the means required, makes sense. It seems plausible to them that other ethical considerations are expendable if sufficient benefit to people can be achieved. To this, Christians can

---

34. John 6:14; cf. 1 John 3:13-18.
35. John 18:20.
36. John 9:4.
37. 1 Cor. 6:19.

only reply, with Paul, that to attribute the view "Let us do evil that good may result" to a Christian is "slanderous."[38] It overlooks both the faithfulness to God and God's ways and the respect for people made in God's image that will not tolerate such an ethics.

So how are we to deal with the different understandings of reality and truth that separate Christians from others in the kosmos? First, we need to recognize that unbelievers cannot be expected to have the same understanding of truth that Christians have. Paul reminds us that: "We have not received the spirit of the kosmos but the Spirit who is from God, that we may understand what God has freely given us. . . . A man without the Spirit does not accept the things that come from the Spirit of God, for they are foolishness to him, and he cannot understand them, because they are spiritually discerned."[39] This suggests that we have two options before us, to be pursued simultaneously: (1) We can help people receive the Spirit of God, and (2) we can translate our language for the benefit of others.

Helping people come to know God and to receive the Spirit of God is of course the better option. There are far more important reasons than ethical agreement for people to know God — including God's glory and their eternal well-being. But in the context of our present discussion, if our ethics are to fully agree, if people are to know the truth about God's intentions for the kosmos, then they must have the same understanding of reality and truth.

Nevertheless, many people will not accept Christ and will reject Christian justifications of ethical positions as foolish. How then are we to communicate with them? Although Paul does not address this explicitly in terms of ethics, he does address essentially the same issue when he confronts the controversy of speaking in tongues. He is happy for people to talk a "strange language" in private, but he is concerned if Christians do so in the presence of unbelievers without regard to its impact on them: "Unless you speak intelligible words with your tongue, how will anyone know what you are saying? You will just be speaking into the air. . . . Will they not say that you are out of your mind?"[40] This is indeed an apt description of the response of many unbelievers today when they hear Christians talking about "*the* truth" and "*the* right way"!

Paul's alternative is to insist on translation and interpretation. If Christians want to communicate the content of something they know through the Spirit of God, then they must use words and concepts that others can under-

38. Rom. 3:8.
39. 1 Cor. 2:12, 14.
40. 1 Cor. 14:9, 23.

stand.[41] In the context of bioethics, this means that we must become thoroughly knowledgeable about the terms in which people think today. We need to understand the approaches to justifying bioethical positions and policies that are most influential in society — approaches such as utilitarian ethics, multiprincipled ethics, and the ultimate postmodern option, autonomy-based ethics. We must develop the ability to argue for our views in the terms of these influential approaches — these kosmos ethics — even though we have arrived at such views through biblically-based Christian analysis.

In doing so, we must avoid two common errors. The first is to operate so exclusively in the realm of kosmos ethics that we start actually formulating our bioethical views in those terms without taking the time to develop explicitly biblical positions we then translate into kosmos language. The problem with this error, which may well afflict many contemporary Christian bioethicists, is that it forces Christians to think primarily in kosmos terms and categories and therefore leads to conclusions that can easily be at odds with a genuinely Christian outlook. The other common error is to be so concerned about translating our bioethics into kosmos language that we forget about or shy away from the first and better strategy for communicating with unbelievers: introducing them to Christ and thereby putting them in touch with the Spirit of God. Seeking opportunities to lead people to Christ and formulating our bioethical views in explicitly biblical-Christian terms must always accompany our bioethical engagement with the kosmos in terms that the kosmos can understand.

Obstacles

Synoptic Gospels

So far, then, we have considered the *challenges* posed by the kosmos as well as the *tasks* God calls us to if we are to make a difference. If we are successfully to engage the kosmos, however, there are obstacles in our path that we must overcome. Some of these obstacles have already been suggested by our description of the kosmos's challenges, including the power that Satan wields over it. Others go beyond these.

The best illustration of such an obstacle in the Synoptic Gospels is the temptation we face to brand worldly people as evil and to undermine their work before it is clear that they truly are evil. Jesus warns his followers about

---

41. 1 Cor. 14:13, 27-28.

this in a parable about a man's field in which weeds have been sown among the wheat plants by his enemy: "The servants asked him, 'Do you want us to go and pull them up?' 'No,' he answered, 'because while you are pulling the weeds, you may root up the wheat with them. . . .' The field is the kosmos. . . . The weeds are the sons of the evil one, and the enemy who sows them is the devil."[42] It is all too easy to become impatient and to be overconfident about our ability to recognize and root out evil without mistakenly hurting current or future believers in the process. People can be misguided but changeable — consider the preconversion and postconversion apostle Paul. They can also be immature — consider the disciple Mark whom Paul refused to bring with him at one point in his ministry. What damage we can do if we are too quick to tear down other people — particularly if they are other biblically-based Christians with whom we differ on particular issues. As previously explained, our primary efforts are to be redemptive — leaving judgment to God.

Writings of John

John, meanwhile, reminds us of how the kosmos itself can become an idol and, therefore, an obstacle. In our desire to have access to the kosmos, it is easy to alter what we say and do in order to win the approval of the kosmos. But John warns, "Do not love the kosmos or anything in the kosmos. If any-one loves the kosmos, the love of the Father is not in that person."[43]

The obstacle here, though, is actually much more than the temptation to seek the world's favor. It is the understandable tendency to go to great lengths to avoid its hatred. "If the kosmos hates you, keep in mind that it hated me first. If you belonged to the kosmos it would love you as its own. As

---

42. Matt. 13:28-29, 38-39.

43. 1 John 2:15. How is it that we are not to love the kosmos according to 1 John 2 — and yet are told in John 3 that God loved the kosmos so much that he sacrificed his son for it? In both passages, the word for love is the same: *agape*. But there is a false kind of love that can seem to Christians or others to be true. Perhaps it is the "love" that moves us to abort a genetically handicapped fetus or to assist the suicide of an ailing adult. However, such apparent compassion is not the true compassion that literally means "suffering with" *(cum + passio)*. Rather, it is yielding to the clamor of our own suffering, which wants to be relieved at all costs. We may even think we act in love, but it is a worldly love — a kosmos love — not a love for God directed sacrificially and redemptively toward the kosmos. Love must first pass the test of honoring God — being in accordance with how God has created and intends the world to be — for loving God is the greatest commandment. The counter-feit love of 1 John 2 involves giving of oneself to gain for oneself; the true love of John 3 in-volves giving of oneself to gain for others.

it is, you do not belong to the kosmos, but I have chosen you out of the kosmos. That is why the kosmos hates you."[44] If we engage the kosmos by speaking God's truth to people and by living an alternative that exposes the fallenness of the kosmos, the kosmos will reject us, as it rejected Jesus Christ.

Nevertheless, it is important to endure such suffering, because in doing so an integrity and power is added to our message that can be obtained in no other way. Jesus understood this as he explained his impending death to his disciples: "I will not speak with you much longer, for the prince of this kosmos is coming. He has no hold on me, but the kosmos must learn that I love the Father and that I do exactly what my Father has commanded me."[45] Not only does such faithful sacrifice enhance the impact of our engagement with the kosmos — it is also the path to eternal life. As Jesus said, those who hate their lives in this kosmos will keep them for eternal life.[46]

It is easy to misstep as we attempt to maneuver around the obstacle of the kosmos's hate. First, we need not assume that it is wrong to defend ourselves or leave a particular encounter with the kosmos if it becomes too intense. Jesus did both at times.[47] We also should not assume that the kosmos's opposition is so strong that no one will listen or respond favorably to what we have to say. Again consider the example of Jesus. While it is true, as John says, that "the kosmos did not recognize him . . . [and] did not receive him," John immediately adds that there were particular individuals who did embrace what he had to say.[48] Such will be our experience as well. When people do respond favorably, we need to avoid the further misstep of thinking that it is simply the result of our skill. Such an attitude will lead to pride or even the incredible burden of thinking we are the world's savior — a role no human can fill. We must always remember that "The Father has sent his Son to be the Savior of the kosmos."[49]

Our task is to be witnesses to who God is and what God intends the kosmos to be. In this role we follow in the steps of Jesus, who said: "For this reason I was born, and for this I came into the kosmos, to testify to the truth."[50] As previously noted, we, like Jesus, are to bring light to the kosmos. Yet again we are mistaken if we think that to bring the light of our witness to

---

44. John 15:18-19. See also John 7:7; 1 John 3:12-13. For other related expressions of opposition, see John 1:9-10; 12:19.

45. John 14:30-31.

46. John 12:25.

47. For example, see John 10:36-40.

48. John 1:10-12; cf. 1 John 4:5-6.

49. 1 John 4:14; cf. John 1:12-13; 17:25.

50. John 18:37.

the kosmos is simply to proclaim our teaching to the kosmos at large, and that a certain number of people will flock to it as insects are drawn to a light. To the contrary, "Light has come into the kosmos, but . . . all who do evil hate the light and will not come into the light for fear that their deeds will be exposed."[51] We need to bring a targeted witness to the kosmos in order to have a significant impact. We must address particular people and structures wherever possible regarding the ways they are at odds with how God would have them live, meanwhile providing them with specific constructive alternatives.

Letters of Paul

When Paul discusses the obstacles before us in our engagement with the kosmos, he, like John, is concerned about various forms of idolatry that can entrap us.[52] His letters warn us in particular of the philosophies and ethics of the day: "See to it that no one takes you captive through hollow and deceptive philosophy, which depends on human traditions and the basic principles of this kosmos rather than on Christ."[53] As noted previously, this does not mean that we cannot use contemporary ways of thinking as tools for communicating with people; it just means that we should not let them become our primary frame of reference. We must not become dependent on them or on anything else in the kosmos. As Paul puts it: "Those who use the things of the kosmos [should live] as if not engrossed in them. For this kosmos in its present form is passing away."[54]

In reaction to the fallenness of the kosmos, it is all too easy to withdraw from relationships with other fallen people. But our tendency to do so is one of the greatest obstacles to making a difference in the kosmos. First, we must draw close to the worst the kosmos has to offer, for those are the very people we most need to reach. Clarifies Paul to the Corinthians: "I have written you in my letter not to associate with sexually immoral people — not at all meaning the people of this kosmos who are immoral, or the greedy and swindlers, or idolaters. In that case you would have to leave this kosmos."[55]

In reaching out, we also must avoid the obstacle of pulling apart into our own personal ministries or our own organizations the way Paul saw people doing in his day — claiming that they were in the Apollos group or the

51. John 3:19-20.
52. 1 Cor. 8:4; 10:14.
53. Col. 2:8.
54. 1 Cor. 7:31.
55. 1 Cor. 5:9-10.

Cephas group or the Paul group.[56] Is our primary loyalty today to a particular denomination, profession, school, organization, or other institution? Or is it to Jesus Christ, his kingdom, and his entire body of people? If it is the latter, then we will work together without arguing among groups or, worse yet, complaining about others when they are not present. Avoiding these obstacles will be part of our distinctive witness. Charges Paul: "Do everything without complaining or arguing, so that you may become blameless and pure, children of God without fault in a crooked and depraved generation, in which you shine like stars in the kosmos."[57]

Resources

Synoptic Gospels

Although the *challenges* posed by the kosmos may seem daunting, the *tasks* before us difficult, and the *obstacles* great, God gives us tremendous *resources* to enable us to make a constructive difference in the kosmos. As the authors of the Synoptic Gospels remind us, the most magnificent of these is the very God of the universe. The devil knows this. That is why he did the best that he could to separate Jesus from God the Father at the very outset of Jesus' engagement with the kosmos. Jesus was in the wilderness, and the devil's first two temptations had failed. So then the devil appealed to something that every follower of God should value extremely highly: the opportunity to have a great impact on the kosmos. "The devil . . . showed him all the kingdoms of the kosmos and their splendor. 'All this I will give you,' he said, 'if you will bow down and worship me.'"[58] The devil knew that if he could separate Jesus from the power and wisdom of God the Father, then Jesus would lose exactly what he needed in order to engage the kosmos effectively.

When that temptation did not work, the devil left him — temporarily. We see evidence of Satan's presence again later, though, when Jesus is talking with his disciples about the way the kosmos will reject him and cause him to suffer. Peter — epitomizing the attitude that successful engagement with the kosmos would mean no suffering — blurts out, "This shall never happen to you!" Jesus rebukes him: "Get behind me, Satan." He chastises him for having a worldly perspective rather than "having in mind the

---

56. 1 Cor. 3:21-22.
57. Phil. 2:14-15.
58. Matt. 4:8-9.

things of God."[59] Jesus then takes advantage of the opportunity to clarify the implications of this encounter for his disciples — though he has Peter in particular in view: "Whoever wants to save his life will lose it, but whoever loses his life for me will find it. What good will it be for a man if he gains the whole kosmos, yet forfeits his soul?"[60] We think that the way to save the kosmos is to go after it in any way that we can with every tool we can obtain. Not so. We must first be committed to God and God's ways. Jesus Christ himself has told us that we must let go of our life and plans and strategies and place him first. Even Satan knows that our ability to make a truly significant difference in the kosmos hinges on the strength of our relationship with God. And even Satan knows that if we become preoccupied with the kosmos for its own sake rather than out of a commitment to glorify God, then Satan has won the battle.

There is a simple way to make sure that we are engaging the kosmos for Christ and not for ourselves. We can ask ourselves if we would be embarrassed if people knew that we were involved in some particular initiative because we worship God. If we would be, we need to ponder the passage in the Gospel of Mark that follows the words just quoted: "If anyone is ashamed of me and my words . . . the Son of Man will be ashamed of him when he comes in his Father's glory."[61] As we endeavor to bring light and truth to the kosmos, we are to act with a particular purpose in mind: "You are the light of the kosmos. . . . Let your light shine before people, that they may see your good deeds and praise your Father in heaven."[62] While there may well be times when we do not broadcast our Christian identity, if we are not identifiably Christian in most of what we do to engage the kosmos, then we are not letting our light shine as Christ has directed, because people cannot know to praise God rather than merely human effort and ability.

Writings of John

If the Synoptic Gospels challenge us to stay close to God as we seek to make a difference, the writings of John fill in greater detail concerning why God is such a crucial resource for our efforts. For example, he is our protection, particularly from Satan. Accordingly, Jesus prays for his followers: "My prayer is

59. Matt. 16:21-23; Mark 8:31-33.
60. Matt. 16:25-26; Mark 8:35-36; Luke 9:24-25.
61. Mark 8:38.
62. Matt. 5:14, 16.

not that you take them out of the kosmos but that you protect them from the evil one."[63] We are deluded if we think that we can do anything substantial in Satan's kosmos and can withstand Satan's attacks in our own strength. It has taken nothing less than the death of Jesus Christ to secure Satan's defeat.[64] But now, if Christ dwells in you, you can rest secure, for "The one who is in you is greater than the one who is in the kosmos."[65] This does not mean that you will not encounter great trials and suffering — the nature of the kosmos insures that you will. But Christ promises to see you through: "In me you may have peace. In this kosmos you will have trouble. But take heart! I have overcome the kosmos."[66]

Knowing this gives us confidence and joy. Although Jesus warns the disciples that they will weep while the kosmos rejoices over his death, he says they are not to worry because they are like pregnant women! Not being bound by the male chauvinist outlook of the kosmos in his day, Jesus is saying that the experience of the pregnant woman going through labor and then birth serves as the perfect example of temporary pain that will give way to great joy.[67] That will be the disciples' experience during Christ's death and resurrection; it is ours in the midst of any defeat we experience in the kosmos as well. God's ways will triumph eventually, and we can start rejoicing in that now.

To confidence and joy, John adds faith and love as potent resources available to Christians desiring to make a significant life-affirming impact on the kosmos. Our first battle with the kosmos is the struggle to break free of its power over us. We must win that before engaging the kosmos further, and faith is the key: "Everyone born of God overcomes the kosmos. This is the victory that has overcome the kosmos, even our faith."[68] As John explains in introducing this verse, such faith is really love directed God-ward, manifested in trusting God enough to live by his commands as we engage the kosmos, rather than trying to make a difference on our own terms.

Christian love, though, is never only God-ward. It is also necessarily directed especially toward other believers with whom we can have a greater constructive impact on the kosmos. The specific purpose for which Jesus asks the Father to protect believers in the kosmos is "so that they may be one."[69]

---

63. John 17:15; cf. 1 John 5:19-20.
64. John 12:31.
65. 1 John 4:4; cf. 5:18-19.
66. John 16:33.
67. John 16:20-22; cf. 17:13.
68. 1 John 5:4.
69. John 17:11.

Apparently the most strategic way that the evil one can neutralize Christians is by separating them and creating antagonism, or at least a lack of connection. When Jesus explicitly looks ahead to future generations of believers, including us, and considers our special need as we engage the kosmos, he prays: "May they be brought to complete unity to let the kosmos know that you sent me and have loved them even as you have loved me."[70] We need to take this prayer seriously and become much more proactive about working together as Christian individuals and organizations, if God's love is to have a major impact on the kosmos.

Letters of Paul

Not surprisingly, Paul approaches our involvement in the kosmos with the same starting point as John. Both insist that our crucial resource is God. That our success depends not on our own worldly abilities but on God comes as great news to most of us, "for God chose the foolish things of the kosmos to shame the wise; God chose the weak things of the kosmos to shame the strong. He chose the lowly things of this kosmos and the despised things — and the things that are not — to nullify the things that are, so that no one may boast before him."[71] If we do have worldly strengths, great. The previous verse does not say that "not any" who are humanly wise or influential or nobly-born become Christians — but rather that "not many" do. For the rest of us, it is encouraging to know that such a background is not a required part of the job description for those who would make a difference in this kosmos for Christ.

Regardless of our natural abilities, we must not rely on them when we do engage the kosmos. We need to be able to say with Paul (who had tremendous human abilities): "This is our boast: Our conscience testifies that we have conducted ourselves in the kosmos . . . not according to worldly wisdom but according to God's grace."[72] Such an approach is essential, for it is through the death of Christ that God is "reconciling the kosmos to himself."[73] When we have "died with Christ to the basic principles of this kosmos" and "continue to live in Christ, rooted and built up in him,"[74] we can remain suffi-

---

70. John 17:23.
71. 1 Cor. 1:27-28.
72. 2 Cor. 1:12.
73. 2 Cor. 5:19.
74. Col. 2:6-7, 20.

ciently free from the kosmos's influence to have a significant impact on the kosmos. We are then ready, in Paul's words, to "fight the good fight."[75]

To protect us in this fight, God gives us a very special resource: the "armor of God."[76] It is crucial that we remember that our struggle "is not against flesh and blood." Otherwise, we will develop clever strategies but be unable to get close enough to the kosmos to implement them effectively without getting undermined or even destroyed in the process. Pieces of armor like righteousness, readiness, faith, and salvation are not optional, they are essential. We should be sure that we are fully armed with them each time we launch an initiative. Moreover, it is worth noting in our present context that the list of armor pieces begins with the "belt of truth" and ends with "the sword of the Spirit, which is the word of God." We need to be shaped and directed by God's truth ourselves, and we must teach its content to one another and to the kosmos.[77]

Before we move on, we should note that before Paul himself is able to move on from this passage, he adds the words "And pray. . . ." Prayer may not be a piece of armor, per se, but it puts us in touch with the person and power of the greatest resource in existence for our work in the world: the God of the universe. If our struggle is indeed with demonic spiritual forces, then how important should we consider prayer to be? Is it only to be occasional — only for some people or certain initiatives? Lest we have any doubt, Paul does not skimp on the superlatives: "And pray in the Spirit on *all* occasions with *all* kinds of prayers and requests. With this in mind, be alert and *always* keep on praying for *all* the saints."[78] Prayer is essential in our walk with God; but, as suggested here, it is equally essential in our work with each other. In fact, praying for one another can be the first step in developing that collaboration that is so essential if our engagement with the kosmos is to be faithful and effective.

Other Letters

To all this counsel, the other New Testament authors add the plea that Christians be wary lest they take for granted their relationship with Christ and not be sufficiently vigilant to guard against the subtle influence of the culture in

75. 1 Tim. 6:7-12.
76. Eph. 6:11-17.
77. According to Col. 2:7-8, such teaching provides the intellectual strength to withstand the worldly thinking that so easily enslaves Christians.
78. Eph. 6:18.

their lives and work. "If they have escaped the corruption of the kosmos by knowing our Lord and Savior Jesus Christ and are again entangled in it and overcome, they are worse off at the end than they were at the beginning."[79] Should we recognize that the kosmos has succeeded in distancing us from God, we can return to God before it is too late. As James puts it: "Come near to God and he will come near to you."[80] But being significantly influenced by the kosmos — "friendship with the kosmos" in James's words — is serious business. It is far more serious than we likely think. To recognize it in our lives, explains James, is cause literally to "grieve, mourn, and wail." Then, using almost exactly the same words as Peter, he says to "humble yourselves before the Lord, and he will lift you up."[81] That is how we "come near to God" — not by going up toward him or by trying to be righteous — but first by going low in repentance and letting God lift us up.

Peter summarizes our challenge in five words, as we face the kosmos: "Prepare your minds for action."[82] Understanding is not opposed to or separate from action. It directs it; it empowers it. Action is not just the realm of the body. It is the realm of the mind and spirit as well. We cannot act effectively until we know what we are trying to accomplish. Do we want God to take us out of the kosmos or take the kosmos out of us? Is our mission to be *in* the kosmos or *into* the kosmos? Do people need to know that we are acting for God or not? Must a substantial portion of every individual's and organization's budget be devoted to collaborative efforts with other Christians? We must think these issues through so that we may act faithfully, and effectively. "Prepare your minds for action." We must appreciate the daunting challenges posed by the kosmos if we are to engage them; we must recognize the difficult tasks at hand if we are to attempt them; we must understand the great obstacles before us if we are to overcome them; but most importantly, we must realize the tremendous resources we have in Christ if we are to make a constructive difference in the kosmos.

---

79. 2 Peter 2:20.
80. James 4:8.
81. James 4:10; 1 Peter 5:6.
82. 1 Peter 1:13-20.

Common Ground and Conflict: The Study of Professional Ethics

David A. Sherwood, M.S.W., Ph.D.

Since worldviews always inform beliefs and beliefs always inform behavior, the integration of faith and practice is a life-long inevitability for all persons, whether they consider themselves religious or not. The only question is how reflective, intentional, and coherent that integration will be.

People in the helping professions tend to use core professional values and codes of ethics as part of the framework of their ethical thinking and integration. Training in professional ethics is a normative part of professional and continuing education. Therefore, the study of professional ethics is a naturally occurring environment in which to engage helping professionals, Christian and non-Christian, in a consciousness-raising process that has integrity for professional education and that allows Christian perspectives to be brought to the table as a legitimate part of the discussion.

A useful strategy is to use the common ground of professional codes of ethics to engage both students and colleagues in a way that integrates worldview assumptions (our own or others') with practice. This essay will explore a simple model of teaching ethics that challenges helping professionals to connect worldviews to ethical theories and principles, to understand the common ground between their own ethical frameworks and professional core values and codes of ethics, and to develop more responsible ways of resolving inevitable tensions between legitimate values at the case level. Social work will be the focus, but the process can be used with the values and codes of ethics of any helping profession. The model can be used effectively in both Christian and non-Christian contexts.

The model is not particularly novel. But it is highly intentional in bringing out the interaction between worldview assumptions, how we understand values and moral responsibility, and the practical application of values and ethics in complex professional judgments in particular cases. The model uses the strategy of taking a core value that all members of the profession presumably affirm on some basic level and find common ground with one another, such as the inherent value of each person. It then unpacks the value in two directions — exploring what supports the common ground and what leads to the unraveling of agreement, and looking at how tensions are resolved when prima facie obligations come into conflict with each other in practice.

First, what kinds of underlying worldview assumptions and ethical theories support the value as commonly understood and agreed on (and what do not)? What are the effects of various worldview assumptions and ethical approaches on how we understand that value? Where and why do professionals start to find their basic agreement unraveling?

Second, we explore the real world of cases, where relevant legitimate values that we still agree on (prima facie obligations) come into tension with one another and we must find ways to prioritize them in the complexities of the situation in which we must make judgments.

Common Ground, Worldviews, and Values: Doesn't Everybody "Just Know" That Persons Have Dignity and Value?

I learned a long time ago that without some sort of common ground it is impossible to communicate, much less reason in hopes of changing minds and hearts. Without it all you can do is fight and see who is the strongest.

I can't help dating myself. I was a freshman at Indiana University in the spring of 1960, in the early days of the Civil Rights Movement. We were hearing of lunchroom sit-ins and Freedom Riders on buses. One evening I spent time at the student commons talking with an older friend of mine from my hometown, Maurice, and someone he had met, a graduate student from Iran named Ali. I was quite impressed. Maurice told me his father was some sort of advisor to the Shah.

The conversation turned to the events in the South, to the ideas of racial integration and social justice. Ali was frankly puzzled and amused that Maurice and I, and at least some other Americans, seemed to think civil rights were worth pursuing. But given that, he found it particularly hard to understand what he thought was the wishy-washy way the thing was being handled. "I don't know why you want to do it," he said, "but if it's so important, why don't you just do it? If I were President of the United States and I wanted integration, I would do it in a week!" "How?" we asked. "Simple. I would just put a soldier with a machine gun on every street corner and say 'Integrate!' If they didn't, I would shoot them."

Now I find his comments believable enough, given what I know of the history of Iran. But back then, naïve freshman that I was, I just couldn't believe he was really saying that. Surely he was putting us on. You couldn't just do that to people. At least not if you were moral! The conversation-debate-argument went on to explore what he really did believe about the innate dignity and value of individual human life and social responsibility. You don't just kill inconvenient people, do you? I would say things like, "Surely you believe that society has a moral responsibility to care for the widows and orphans, the elderly, disabled, the emotionally disturbed." Incredibly (to me at the time), Ali's basic response was not to give an inch, but to question *my* beliefs and values instead. He said, "On the contrary. You keep talking about reason and morality. I'll tell you what's unreasonable and immoral. The rational person would say that the truly *immoral* thing is to take resources away from the strong and productive to give to the weak and useless. Useless members of society such as the disabled and mentally retarded should be eliminated, not maintained." Being a sensitive man, he would prefer that the methods be "humane," but he really did mean "eliminated."

It finally sunk into my freshman mind that what we were disagreeing about was not facts or logic, but the belief systems we were using to interpret or assign meaning to the facts. Ali was a thoroughly secular man — he had left Islam and any concept of a God behind. He believed that the material universe is the extent of reality and that self-preservation is the only given motive and goal. If I were to accept his assumptions about the nature of the universe, then his logic was flawless and honest. The only thing of importance left to discuss would be the most effective means to gain and keep power and the most expedient way to use it.

In this encounter I was shaken loose from my naïve assumption that "everybody knows" the individual person has innate dignity and value. I understood clearly that unless you believed in a Creator or some transcendent basis of value, the notion that all persons are equal is, indeed, *not* self-evident. The Nazi policies of eugenics and the "final solution" to the "Jewish problem" make a kind of grimly honest (almost inevitable) sense if you believe in the materialist worldview.

The "Is-Ought" Dilemma

Not long afterward I was to encounter this truth much more cogently expressed in the writings of C. S. Lewis. In *The Abolition of Man* he points out that both the "religious" and the "secular" walk by faith if they try to move from descriptive observations of fact to any sort of value statement or ethical imperative. He says, "From propositions about fact alone no *practical* conclusion can ever be drawn. 'This will preserve society' [let's assume this is a factually true statement] cannot lead to 'Do this' [a moral and practical injunction] except by the mediation of [the value statement] 'Society ought to be preserved.'"[1] "Society ought to be preserved" is a moral imperative which no amount of facts alone can prove or disprove. Even the idea of "knowing facts" involves basic assumptions (or faith) about the nature of the universe and human minds. The secular person tries to cloak faith by substituting words like "natural," "necessary," "progressive," "scientific," "rational," or "functional" for "good," but the question always remains — "For what end?" and "Why?" And the answer to this question always smuggles in values.

Even resorting to "instincts" such as self-preservation can tell us nothing about what we (or others) *ought* to do. Lewis says:

> We grasp at useless words: we call it the "basic," or "fundamental," or "primal," or "deepest" instinct. It is of no avail. Either these words conceal a value judgment passed *upon* the instinct and therefore not derivable *from* it, or else they merely record its felt intensity, the frequency of its operation, and its wide distribution. If the former, the whole attempt to base value upon instinct has been abandoned: if the latter, these observations about the quantitative aspects of a psychological event lead to no practical conclusion. It is the old dilemma. Either the premises already concealed an imperative or the conclusion remains merely in the indicative.[2]

This is called the "Is-Ought" dilemma. Facts, even when attainable, never have any practical or moral implications until they are interpreted through the grid of some sort of value assumptions. "Is" does not lead to "Ought" in any way that has moral bindingness, obligation, or authority until its relationship to relevant values is understood. And you can't get the values directly from the "Is." It always comes down to the question — what is the source and authority of the "Ought" that is claimed or implied?

1. C. S. Lewis, *The Abolition of Man* (New York: Macmillan, 1947), p. 43.
2. Lewis, *Abolition of Man*, p. 49.

Common ground, then, might seem to be very hard to come by. Spiritually and philosophically, it often is. Practically, however, it is not so hard to find as we sometimes might think. And this gives us the opportunity to explore the spiritual and philosophical. Regardless of what might be the relativistic and materialistic logical implications of the worldviews many hold, we nevertheless find it difficult to be thoroughly relativistic and materialistic when push comes to shove. At some point, most of us find ourselves wanting to say, "No, *that* is really wrong" or "*That* is really good." And we don't mean simply that we find it to be a mere personal preference.

Professional Codes of Ethics as "Common Ground"

Professional codes of ethics, such as the social work Code of Ethics, refer to core values such as the inherent value of every person, the importance of social justice, and the obligation to fight against oppression. It is a fair question to ask where those values come from and what gives them moral authority and obligation. Christians do not only affirm these values; we have a worldview that gives them meaning and authority.

For example, the social work Code of Ethics enumerates six core values and their related ethical principles:

1. **Service.** *Ethical Principle:* Social workers' primary goal is to help people in need and to address social problems.
2. **Social Justice.** *Ethical Principle:* Social workers challenge social injustice.
3. **Dignity and Worth of the Person.** *Ethical Principle:* Social workers respect the inherent dignity and worth of the person.
4. **Importance of Human Relationships.** *Ethical Principle:* Social workers recognize the central importance of human relationships.
5. **Integrity.** *Ethical Principle:* Social workers behave in a trustworthy manner.
6. **Competence.** *Ethical Principle:* Social workers practice within their areas of competence and develop and enhance their professional expertise.[3]

This is common ground. At the level of core values such as these and their related ethical principles, Christians can wholeheartedly affirm their

3. National Association of Social Workers, *Code of Ethics* (Annapolis Junction, Md.: NASW Press, 1996).

professional identity and find common ground with their non-Christian colleagues.

The exploration of core professional values and professional codes of ethics provides the ideal context for making a difference in creating a life-affirming impact in professional education, continuing education, and relationships with professional colleagues. It can help overcome stereotypes regarding difference, affirming what we hold in common. It can clarify the nature of our actual differences and conflicts, facilitating growth-producing dialogue.

The Basic Strategy

The basic strategy of exploring ethical common ground and the nature of the conflicts we have is one which I have evolved in the process of teaching professional values and ethics to social work students at both the undergraduate and graduate levels. I try to teach values and ethics in a way that respects and integrates both my own Christian and professional values and those of my students, colleagues, and clients, who may disagree with me in many ways. Maintaining our own integrity while respecting the integrity of others is an essential Christian value as well as professional value. I will outline the basic strategy and then elaborate on it a bit.

1. Find common ground in core professional values and their related ethical principles articulated in our professional code of ethics. An example would be the inherent value of every person.
2. Introduce the nature of ethical dilemmas, which by definition involve conflicts and tensions between legitimate prima facie values, principles, or duties that somehow must be prioritized in the case at hand. Examples would be self-determination versus protection from harm, freedom versus well-being.
3. Establish a basis for discussion and mutual respect under conditions of disagreement by clarifying that the further we move from the core values through related principles to applications of judgment in specific cases, the more conscientious persons will disagree.
4. Explore both common ground and conflict through the discussion of the application of professional ethics to a particular ethical dilemma or case.

1. Find common ground in core professional values and their related ethical principles articulated in our professional code of ethics.

Professional codes of ethics typically articulate core professional values and related ethical principles at a level of generality that Christians should have no difficulty agreeing with and strongly endorsing. In fact, these core values typically express Judeo-Christian values or the common human moral intuitions which C. S. Lewis once described as "The Way" or "The Tao."[4]

In the social work Code of Ethics, a central value relating to the affirmation of life is the "dignity and worth of the person." The broad ethical principle the code articulates based on this value is "Social workers respect the inherent dignity and worth of the person." Another important value is "social justice," and its accompanying ethical principle "Social workers challenge social injustice."[5]

We should try very hard to make it clear to our students, colleagues, and clients that we affirm the core values and ethical principles of our profession. And we should make it very clear that, far from conflicting with professional values, our Christian faith undergirds that affirmation.

2. Introduce the nature of ethical dilemmas, which by definition involve conflicts and tensions between legitimate prima facie values, principles, or duties that somehow must be prioritized in the case at hand.

I tell my students that all ethical dilemmas involve conflicts or tensions between more than one legitimate prima facie value, principle, or duty. If there is only one value at stake or one "good" value and one "bad" value, we may have a character problem in summoning up the courage to do what we know we should do, but we don't have an ethical dilemma. A prima facie value or duty is one which we recognize as a legitimate moral obligation "on its face," such as telling the truth, maintaining confidentiality, and protecting people from harm. Codes of ethics are full of these. So are the Ten Commandments and the Sermon on the Mount. From time to time prima facie values come into tension with each other and practical action forces us to make some sort of prioritization or resolution. This is an ethical dilemma. When we encounter and resolve (at least provisionally) an ethical dilemma, it does not mean (necessarily) that we have abandoned or ignored any of the values that we subscribe to. It is simply the case that, in this fallen and finite world, "you cannot maximize all values simultaneously" (Sherwood's Maxim). The choice

---

4. Lewis, *Abolition of Man.*
5. NASW, *Code of Ethics,* p. 5.

to do one thing *always* means giving up or having less of something else. And that something else may be a very good thing. Serious choices are usually very costly ones.

A classic example in social work and in other helping professions is the tension that may develop between freedom and well-being. Under the heading "Social Workers' Ethical Responsibilities to Clients" is found section 1.02, "Self-Determination," which reads:

> Social workers respect and promote the right of clients to self-determination and assist clients in their efforts to identify and clarify their goals. Social workers may limit clients' right to self-determination when, in the social workers' professional judgment, clients' actions or potential actions pose a serious, foreseeable, and imminent risk to themselves or others.[6]

This is a clear attempt to articulate an important dimension of freedom, but even here there is a recognition that the prima facie good of freedom cannot be absolutized without consideration of the prima facie good of well-being, both for the client and for others. This ethical standard recognizes two legitimate values and the necessity for professionals to make judgments which take them both into account but which, because of the tension involved in a particular case, will always involve some abridgment of one or both of the values. What does it mean to "limit clients' right to self-determination"? What constitutes "serious, foreseeable, and imminent risk"? How bad does it have to be before it justifies interfering with another person's self-determination?

Thus codes of ethics often recognize this inevitable tension between legitimate prima facie values and may even offer some guidance in prioritization. But they do not presume to resolve them prescriptively. Judgment is always required. The National Association of Social Workers (NASW) Code of Ethics articulates this very clearly. "Core values, and the principles that flow from them, must be balanced within the context and complexity of the human experience."[7] "The *Code* offers a set of values, principles, and standards to guide decision making and conduct when ethical issues arise. It does not provide a set of rules that prescribe how social workers should act in all situations. Specific applications of the *Code* must take into account the context in which it is being considered and the possibility of conflicts among the *Code*'s values, principles, and standards."[8]

---

6. NASW, *Code of Ethics*, p. 7.
7. NASW, *Code of Ethics*, p. 1.
8. NASW, *Code of Ethics*, p. 8.

3. Establish a basis for discussion and mutual respect under conditions of disagreement by clarifying that the further we move from the core values through related principles to applications of judgment in specific cases, the more conscientious persons will disagree.

I try to help students understand that even when they agree with each other on core values and ethical principles, they may do so for different reasons. Further, even when they agree on the reasons they will inevitably find themselves disagreeing with each other more and more as they move from the fundamental level of presuppositions and worldview to principles, to rules that guide the application of principles, and to the specific decisions and actions required by case situations. This is important for Christians and non-Christians alike to understand. It provides a basis for mutual respect under conditions of conscientious disagreement by helping them not to expect more consensus than is appropriate. We agree that we want to achieve social justice in regard to poverty, but we may legitimately disagree over what will effectively contribute to that goal and which values we are willing to put at greater risk in the process of seeking it.

I utilize the image of a pyramid and then borrow language from Arthur Holmes of "bases," "principles," "rules," and "cases."[9] If we visualize a pyramid, we can think of the bottom section as representing the "Bases" or fundamental worldview assumptions behind our values and ethics.

I explain the concept that worldview assumptions are inevitable and universal among humans as we attempt to make sense of the world around us and our place in it, regardless of the particular content of the assumptions — religious or secular, explicit or implicit. Religious or secular, worldviews give faith-based answers to a set of four ultimate and grounding questions, posed this way by Middleton and Walsh:

- **Where are we?** What is the nature of reality, the universe we find ourselves in?
- **Who are we?** What is the nature and task of human beings?
- **What's wrong?** How do we understand and account for evil and brokenness?
- **What's the remedy?** How can we find a path through our brokenness to wholeness?[10]

9. Arthur Holmes, *Ethics: Approaching Moral Decisions* (Downers Grove, Ill.: InterVarsity Press, 1985).

10. J. Richard Middleton and Brian J. Walsh, *Truth Is Stranger Than It Used to Be: Biblical Faith In a Postmodern Age* (Downers Grove, Ill.: InterVarsity Press, 1995).

I ask students to scrutinize all theories and interpretations on the basis of what implicit or explicit assumptions they make regarding these basic questions. Christians will find themselves with the highest level of agreement with each other at this level. On the other hand, Christians and non-Christians may *not* find themselves at the highest level of agreement at this level, an important point that we can come back to and explore later.

The next level up the pyramid can represent "Principles" or core values that rest on the worldview assumptions (or faith) below. It is at this level that Christian and non-Christian professionals will have the highest level of agreement with each other. This is the level of the "exceptionless absolutes"[11] of love and justice for the Christian, and for the core values such as the worth and dignity of every person for the Christian and non-Christian alike.

The next level up the pyramid is that of "Rules," deontological and utilitarian rules that guide the application of the principles to various areas of life. Deontological rules are statements of moral obligation or "oughts" perceived to be morally binding, such as truth-telling, confidentiality, non-exploitation. The Ethical Standards of the social work Code of Ethics constitute such rules or guidelines. For Christians, the Ten Commandments, the Sermon on the Mount, and other teachings of Scripture would fall here. It is important to realize that these rules are prima facie goods, but they cannot be absolutized independently of their interaction with one another. This is why rules, even God's rules, can never provide us with prescriptive formulas that remove the necessity and responsibility for making moral judgments in given situations.

Utilitarian rules, I would argue, are ancillary to deontological rules and point to prediction and evaluation of consequences in regard to the achievement of what must ultimately be a deontologically justified goal or good. From a purely utilitarian perspective actions are good if they achieve the "good" result. Ends, not means, are what ultimately count from a utilitarian perspective. But it is the "Is-Ought" dilemma I referred to earlier — in order to define the "good end" utilitarianism always has to smuggle in at least one "ought" that cannot be pragmatically derived.

Christians and non-Christians will tend to have a high level of agreement regarding the basic moral rules as they are embodied in professional codes of ethics. However, they will tend to disagree on what justifies the basic rules and on what basis they would be prioritized. This is where the "bases" — worldview assumptions — make themselves felt.

At the top of the pyramid the bases, principles, and rules are applied to specific situations or cases. It is here that the rules come into tension or con-

11. Holmes, *Ethics*.

flict with one another and yet some judgment must be made and some action taken. It is here that the level of conflict is the greatest and most evident, even among those who agree on everything up to this point. Why is this?

1. *Limited and varying grasp of the moral issues at stake.* Life is temptingly much simpler if we can be content to reduce the terms in the moral equation. Decision and action are much simpler if abortion is *only* about privacy, a woman's right to make choices regarding her own life and body. *Or* if it is *only* about the protection of life, including fetal life at any stage of development. Honest ethical analysis involves trying to identify *all* the moral issues at stake and giving them their rightful place at the table. This includes big issues that we are not likely to find easy (or any) resolution for, such as "What does it mean to be a 'person'?" "What does it mean to have a 'right to life' and what is that right based on?" "What limits, if any, are there to personal autonomy and freedom?"

2. *Limited and varying grasp of the relevant facts.* While values can't be derived from facts alone (the "Is-Ought" dilemma), facts can and do inform our understanding of what is at stake in moral issues and our practical actions. We live and act under the reality that our knowledge of the relevant facts is always going to be limited, but that we are under obligation to bring the best knowledge we can muster to bear on the moral judgments we have to make in a specific case. We are fallen and finite, limited in time, capacity, and access. What effects, for example, will legally mandating parental consent for a minor to receive an abortion have on the number of abortions, the children themselves, parent-child relationships?

3. *Limited and varying grasp of the actual intended and unintended consequences of a given course of action, program, or policy.* This is an extension of the previous point about our limited understanding of the relevant facts. We say, legitimately I think, that ethical judgments and actions should at least take into consideration their practical consequences and that some results are "better" than others. "What is going to happen if I do this, and is that better than the alternatives?" Considerations of consequences in ethical decision making often sound "factual," "pragmatic," or "utilitarian" on the surface, and in certain ways they are. However, it is important to realize that what we are thinking of in terms of "results" or "consequences" of various possible courses of action can never be more than "best guess" *predictions* at the time we are trying to make an ethical judgment. I may think I know, but I may be tragically wrong. Or I may be painfully aware of how limited my ability is to anticipate the conse-

quences of the various choices in front of me, yet choose and act I must. Actual consequences include both those I intend and those that I do not intend, but which nonetheless follow. Will, for example, providing condoms to teenagers foster promiscuity, decrease teen pregnancy, slow the spread of AIDS, or (as is quite possible) all three?

4. *Differences regarding prioritization of legitimate prima facie values.* It is on this level of cases that we are always having to make judgments or take actions that inevitably represent a prioritizing of values. This is Sherwood's Maxim again: "You can't maximize all values simultaneously," and its corollary, "So you have to know how to weigh your choices as you come as close as you can." Does personal autonomy and freedom trump all other values, as our culture tends to believe? How does individual freedom weigh compared with justice or the common good? My good versus the good of others? Whether we like it or not, every actual policy, program, or practice intervention we can conceive of is a sort of "compromise" that represents a balancing of competing legitimate (but not always equally important) values. We want, for example, to help the "truly needy," especially children, but how do we do that in a way that does not foster dependency?

5. *Not only finite, but fallen.* From the Christian perspective, the human predicament is not simply one of limits, but fundamental distortion — we are not only finite, we are fallen. This inevitably affects our ethical thinking and behavior, leading even those who share the same worldview, affirm the same principles and rules, and accept the same facts to find themselves in disagreement. Our self-centeredness, fears, and anger distort our perception and judgment. The apostle Peter was sincere and meant well, but he denied Jesus three times.

All of these considerations help us to find a basis for understanding and respecting those who disagree with us — our brothers and sisters in Christ, our professional colleagues, our clients, and others. These considerations also suggest areas for us to discuss and explore with one another as we seek to understand both common ground and where we conflict.

4. Explore both common ground and conflict through the discussion of the application of professional ethics to a particular ethical dilemma or case.

The discussion of cases provides a professionally legitimate opportunity to explore what resources we can bring to bear to help us make ethically grounded decisions. Discussion of cases using professional codes of ethics allows us to work back through the levels of the pyramid: What are the relevant rules? Where do factual knowledge and consequentialist calculations and predictions fit into the picture? How do theoretical frameworks shape our perceptions and interpretations? What fundamental core values and moral principles are we attempting to bring to life? What worldview assumptions about the nature of the world and persons inform and guide our approach to the issues?

A Brief Example:
"The Inherent Dignity and Worth of the Person"

Bioethics is full of relevant examples of ethical dilemmas for the helping professional. I will briefly discuss one to illustrate the use of the study of professional ethics to help professionals deepen their understanding of their own principles and practice and those of others.

For example, both the issue of abortion itself and how professionals handle their ethical convictions concerning abortion in practice with clients and colleagues reflect important concerns that any competent professional must address. I will not try to cover these considerations in depth, only enough to give a feel for the approach that I have been discussing.

Why Is Abortion a Problem?

After laying some of the groundwork discussed above, I might ask students why abortion presents moral dilemmas to individuals and to professionals. I may have some students who do not think abortion represents a moral dilemma (either because they see no reason why it might be wrong or no reason why it might ever be justified). I then ask them to at least speculate why other people might see it as a moral problem. It is usually not very difficult to get out on the table some of the moral issues that they think might be at stake in abortion: individual freedom and autonomy; the nature of life and personhood; protection of human life; emotional, physical, and financial well-being; prevention of harm to women; equal access to treatment.

Core Values in the Code of Ethics

I then ask them to identify elements of the social work Code of Ethics that might relate to some of the issues they have identified. Core values and ethical principles that quickly emerge include "Service" — Social workers' primary goal is to help people in need and to address social problems; "Social Justice" — Social workers challenge social injustice; and "Dignity and Worth of the Person" — Social workers respect the inherent dignity and worth of the person.

Worldviews and Ethical Concepts

Helping, social justice, and the dignity and worth of each person are important but broad and complex concepts. If time permits, we may explore alternative worldview assumptions and how they do or do not support such concepts, or if they do, how they might give the concepts different content.

For example, evolutionary materialism, utilitarianism, libertarian individualism, and rational liberal humanism lead to very different notions of what constitutes "social justice." I point out that "fairness" is to some extent defined by and always inseparable from what we believe about the nature of persons, rights, moral obligation, and "the good." If we believe in karma and reincarnation, we might believe that a caste system with Brahmans and untouchables is just and that it would be wrong to interfere with it. If we believe that God has ordained a hierarchy of social positions and sovereignly placed people in it, we might believe that the divine right of certain families to be kings and others to be slaves is just. If we believe that might makes right, then "success" is just.

What Does It Mean to Be a Person?

The social work value of the "dignity and worth of the person" is always worth some exploration. What does it mean to be a person? What are the qualifications? How do you achieve that status and can you lose it? Where do "dignity and worth" come from and what do they consist of? Many people today associate personhood with certain capacities of rational self-consciousness, purposive action, and emotional response. However, they may not have thought through the logical implications of this, particularly regarding the status of the unborn, infants, the comatose, the severely mentally disabled. It can be very helpful to unpack the implications of this definition. Even if some students are willing to accept the implication, for example, that even infants do not measure up to this definition strictly and may be eligible for selective elimination, at least they have taken intellectual ownership of their beliefs. Many will be prompted to reconsider their beliefs.

I sometimes use a handout based on Robert Wennberg's book *Life in the*

Balance: Exploring the Abortion Controversy[12] to facilitate discussion of the meaning of personhood and what makes human life of value and deserving of protection. This is not because I necessarily agree with him in all the particulars of his conclusions (I do not), but because he does a good job of laying out the issues and the implications of some of the different worldview assumptions. I label the handout "An Example of a Christian Ethical Analysis" and include some materials from Gilbert Meilaender's *Bioethics: A Primer for Christians*[13] to illustrate that not all Christians come to exactly the same conclusions. I also encourage students to read selected articles representing a variety of points of view concerning what constitutes personhood and is the basis for the "dignity and worth of the person."

What Does the Code of Ethics Say?

We then examine the social work Code of Ethics for relevant ethical standards which attempt to explicate the core values in regard to more specific ethical responsibilities to clients, colleagues, practice settings, the profession, and the broader society. Here we begin to see more clearly how legitimate prima facie moral obligations may come into tension with one another in case situations and require some principled means of prioritization. For example:

Section 1.01: Commitment to Clients says:

Social workers' primary responsibility is to promote the well-being of clients. In general, clients' interests are primary. However, social workers' responsibility to the larger society or specific legal obligations, may on limited occasions supersede the loyalty owed clients, and clients should be so advised.[14]

Section 1.02: Self-Determination says:

Social workers respect and promote the right of clients to self-determination and assist clients in their efforts to identify and clarify their goals. Social workers may limit clients' right to self-determination when, in the social workers' professional judgment, clients' actions or

---

12. Robert N. Wennberg, *Life in the Balance: Exploring the Abortion Controversy* (Grand Rapids: Eerdmans, 1985).

13. Gilbert Meilaender, *Bioethics: A Primer for Christians* (Grand Rapids: Eerdmans, 1996).

14. NASW, *Code of Ethics*, p. 7.

potential actions pose a serious, foreseeable, and imminent risk to themselves or others.[15]

Section 1.06: Conflicts of Interest says, in part:

(a) Social workers should be alert to and avoid conflicts of interest that interfere with the exercise of professional discretion and impartial judgment. Social workers should inform clients when a real or potential conflict of interest arises and take reasonable steps to resolve the issue in a manner that makes the clients' interests primary and protects clients' interest to the greatest extent possible. In some cases, protecting clients' interests may require termination of the professional relationship with proper referral of the client.

(b) Social workers should not take unfair advantage of any professional relationship or exploit others to further their personal, religious, political, or business interests.[16]

It is important to help students see how these guidelines have prima facie validity but that in practice they can come into tension with one another, requiring resolution.

Using Principles to Prioritize Prima Facie Ethical Obligations: A Social Work Example

At this point, I show how some of the best known and respected social work writers on ethics have tried to deal with the issue of recognizing and resolving tensions between prima facie ethical obligations. A primary example would be Frederic Reamer, chairperson of the committee that produced the 1996 revision of the NASW Code of Ethics, and author of several books on social work ethics, including *Ethical Dilemmas in Social Service*[17] and *Current Controversies in Social Work Ethics: Case Examples*.[18] I like to use Reamer because he is

15. NASW, *Code of Ethics*, p. 7.
16. NASW, *Code of Ethics*, p. 9.
17. Frederic Reamer, *Ethical Dilemmas in Social Service*, 2nd ed. (New York: Columbia University Press, 1993).
18. Frederic Reamer, *Current Controversies in Social Work Ethics: Case Examples* (Annapolis Junction, Md.: NASW Press, 1998). See also Frank M. Loewenberg and Ralph Dolgoff, *Ethical Decisions for Social Work Practice*, 5th ed. (Itaska, Ill.: F. E. Peacock, 1996).

thoughtful, sophisticated about both ethics and practice, well-balanced, and quite clear in the way he lays out his thinking and the principles behind it.

Reamer clearly rejects complete relativism. "If one believes that conclusions concerning ethical values and guidelines reflect only *opinions* about the rightness and wrongness of specific actions and that objective standards do not exist, there is no reason to even attempt to determine whether certain actions are *in fact* right or wrong. One opinion would be considered as acceptable as another."[19] He opts for "reason" as providing a sufficient basis to derive moral obligation and even to help rank obligations. Building on Gewirth, Reamer starts with the concept of "personhood" as "agency." What are the logical requirements or necessary goods in order to take purposive action? All "responsible persons" have a "generic right" to the essential conditions to act as persons (make free choices and act). These necessary conditions or goods, then, are freedom and basic well-being. And if we want this for ourselves we are logically required to want and respect this for other persons (Gewirth's version of the Golden Rule). From this premise Reamer develops basic rules or criteria for resolving conflicts between prima facie duties which happen to comport very well with Western liberal democratic thinking. Freedom is the highest value, but it can't be exercised without basic well-being. So, for example:

1. **Basic goods take precedence over other goods.** Rules against basic harms to the necessary preconditions of action (life, shelter, health, food, mental equilibrium) take precedence over rules against harms to nonsubtractive goods (lying, revealing confidential material) or additive goods (recreation, education, wealth).

2. **The individual well-being of others takes precedence over my personal freedom.** Another person's right to basic well-being takes precedence over my right to freedom.

3. **An individual's freedom takes precedence over that individual's own well-being.** My freedom (assuming voluntary, informed choice) takes precedence over my own well-being.

4. **The obligation to obey laws, rules freely consented to, normally takes precedence over individual freedom.** Rules and regulations to which I have voluntarily and freely consented originally override my right to act voluntarily and freely in a manner which conflicts with these laws and policies.

5. **The basic well-being of persons takes precedence over laws, rules, and regulations.** An individual's right to basic well-being may override laws,

19. Reamer, *Ethical Dilemmas*, p. 55.

regulations, and arrangements of voluntary associations in cases of conflict.

6. **The obligation to prevent basic harm and promote public goods takes precedence over property rights.** The obligation to prevent harms to basic well-being of persons such as starvation and to promote public goods such as housing, education, and public assistance overrides individuals' rights to retain all of their property (justifying taxation for the public good).[20]

Reamer then goes on to illustrate the application of the Code of Ethics and his principles to complex case situations in which prima facie obligations come into conflict and must be resolved. He is properly clear on the fact that no principles, rules, or guidelines can provide unambiguous, undebatable solutions to moral dilemmas, but that they can give us invaluable help. I can discuss with students his excellent example of ethical analysis based on worldview assumptions, core values and ethical principles, area rules, and the principled prioritization required by application to hard cases. I can also legitimately discuss alternate worldview assumptions and principles which might be utilized to define and prioritize these social work core values, including Christian ones.

The Challenge of Ethical Integrity and Helping Practice

I want students to understand that no one is "objective" regarding the meaning of personhood and the nature and value of human life. I want them to know that we all have worldview assumptions that frame our perceptions of these issues, that these beliefs will influence how we practice with clients and colleagues, and that we have both a personal and professional ethical obligation to handle these values issues with integrity. One of the implications is that appropriate handling of personal values is not just an issue for Christians, but that all professionals face essentially the same challenge. All of us must learn how to have integrity with our own values while avoiding exploiting our professional position to "impose" our values on clients especially, but also colleagues.

So, we talk about what that kind of integrity might require of us, no matter where we are on the ideological or religious spectrum. My Christian students need to understand that they are not abandoning their faith when

20. Reamer, *Ethical Dilemmas*, pp. 62-65.

they appropriately refrain from exploiting their professional relationships with clients for purposes of evangelism. My non-Christian students need to understand that the Christian students are committed to the same ethical standards of practice they are, and that they themselves can be as easily tempted as anyone else to exploit their professional relationships with clients to "impose" their own moral, spiritual, or political agendas. Actually, they can perhaps be tempted more so, if they naively believe that imposing values is a problem that religious people have but which they are above. Both my Christian and non-Christian students need to understand that they don't solve the issue of misusing values, spirituality, and religion by simply avoiding the subjects with their clients. Honesty and sensitivity to what is relevant to the client and the situation must prevail. Both Christian and non-Christian students need to understand that there may come a time in work with certain clients that the clients' goals are such that the social worker cannot in good conscience pursue them with the clients. At that point (if not before), social workers may need to clarify the implications of informed consent so clients can make their own choices, possibly including referral to another worker.

I hope that my students and I will have a better understanding of ethical analysis and decision making. I hope we clearly see the value and limits of codes of ethics, that they provide helpful guidance but never prescriptive answers regarding genuine dilemmas. I hope that we will understand our own values and the implications of those values. I hope that we will understand and respect other conscientious professionals who are trying to maximize legitimate values when they come into real tension with one another. I want us all to be able to find and affirm our common ground and to understand as well as possible what is at stake where we are in real conflict.

Persons of Character Who Act in Love and Justice

But understanding will only take us so far. When all is said and done, our morality (or lack of it) depends much more on *who* we are than what we know or what procedures we use to analyze ethical dilemmas. We must become persons who have taken on the mind and character of Christ as new creations. God intends no less than to "grow us up" in a way that fits with who he has made us and what we have made ourselves. Morally, this means "growing up" is measured by nothing less than the righteousness of God. That righteousness was not encompassed by the law but was embodied in the person of Jesus Christ. Jesus made moral judgments and took action in the context of human and physical limitations just like we do, yet he revealed God's character of love and justice in action. Jesus was led by the law; indeed he "fulfilled" it (Matt. 5:17). But his judgments and actions were not legalistic. Instead they integrated and reconciled the sometimes conflicting demands of God's law through being fully led by God's Spirit, embodying God's very character in human terms.

It appears that the heart of Christian morality and ethics is not found in laws and rules but in the nature and character of a person, God-in-the-flesh, Jesus Christ. The law and rules may be schoolmasters or disciplinarians (see Gal. 3:23-25), but if they don't lead us to the Word made flesh they will kill us. Christian ethical teaching always comes down to "Be like Jesus" rather than "Follow this rule, no matter what."

Good professional ethical judgments are most likely to be achieved by persons possessing both professional competence (including ethical competence) and virtuous character. May we become persons of character who act in love and justice, our choices guided by the Spirit of Christ.

The Vertical Context:
Prayer and Bioethics

Dónal P. O'Mathúna, Ph.D.

Christians seeking to make a difference in their culture know they need help from God. But how should that help be sought? What should Christians do to ensure that God is at the center of their attempts to make a difference?

A Christian's prayer life presents direct insight into his or her level of dependence on the Lord. In my own life, I have struggled with how to make sure that what I am doing is what God would want me to do. How do I know if the things I say to my students, colleagues, and others are what God wants me to say? How do I know that what I write is what God wants written? How do I know that how I treat this person in front of me is how God would have me treat her? How do I know whether God would approve or disapprove of this policy we have to vote on? The answers to these questions cannot come unless the questions are brought before God in prayer. All Christians need vital prayer lives, in which God's perspective on all these issues is sought consistently and regularly.

Scripture provides excellent examples of godly men and women seeking to make a difference in their world. This chapter is divided into two sections. The first half will use Psalm 141 to develop some strategies for prayer directed in a vertical direction: towards God himself. The second half will look at how prayer can make a difference horizontally: directed towards others in our lives. Although this division is somewhat artificial, it provides an approach which will help keep our prayer lives balanced.

The Vertical Dimension

Psalm 141 opens:

> O Lord, I call upon You; hasten to me!
> Give ear to my voice when I call to You!

First of all, Christians need to reflect on whether they turn to God about these issues at all. God really cares about what is going on "down here." He certainly wants people to come to know him, and he wants people to worship him, but sometimes it is less clear if he cares about the policies adopted at various institutions. Christians firmly believe it makes a difference to God whether assisted suicide is legalized, or abortion. But what about the financial policies at our organizations? We may seriously doubt that God could be concerned about the many other, "lesser" policies at our institutions. In that case, we are unlikely to pray about how those policies are developed or implemented.

Christians should believe that God is concerned about all these decisions. He cares about all aspects of people's lives. Paul encouraged the people to pray for their political leaders (1 Tim. 2:1-2). The policies implemented at every level are based on values and beliefs, some of which help promote or demote Christian values. God's help should be sought for discernment on these issues. He promises to give direction in all aspects of life.

> May my prayer be counted as incense before You;
> The lifting up of my hands as the evening offering. (Ps. 141:2)

David here refers to the ceremonial practices of the time.[1] Every morning and every evening, the priests offered incense and sacrifices at the altar. The term used for offering is *minchath*, which was used of the gratitude offering, not a blood offering (which is rendered by *zebach*). David compares his prayer to the offerings made to God. These were made daily, regardless of what else was occurring. They were offered in complete humility, knowing that these were an important way to express one's dependence on and praise for Yahweh. These were offered in an air of thankfulness for all that God had already done. Christians should examine themselves and ask if they, like David, pray with humility, thanking God for what he has already done, and knowing, by faith, that he will bring about what is needed in a particular situation.

---

1. Frank E. Gaebelein, ed., *The Expositor's Bible Commentary* (Grand Rapids: Zondervan, 1991), 5:846.

> Set a guard, O Lord, over my mouth;
> Keep watch over the door of my lips.
> Do not incline my heart to any evil thing,
> To practice deeds of wickedness with men who do iniquity;
> And do not let me eat of their delicacies. (vv. 3-4)

David prays for direction from God. He prays against the temptations that he knows will come his way. And most notably, he prays against his tongue! He realizes, as James later states more directly, that

> the tongue is a small part of the body, and yet it boasts of great things. Behold, how great a forest is set aflame by such a small fire! And the tongue is a fire, the very world of iniquity; the tongue is set among our members as that which defiles the entire body, and sets on fire the course of our life, and is set on fire by hell. . . . But no one can tame the tongue; it is a restless evil and full of deadly poison. . . . My brethren, these things ought not to be this way. (James 3:5-10)

We need to acknowledge and confess our weaknesses and pray against giving in to temptation. The word "delicacies" vividly describes the world system and all it offers. It is often not blatantly evil and repugnant. Just as Satan can disguise himself as an angel of light (2 Cor. 11:14), the ways of the world are often more attractive, more comfortable, easier, less controversial, and sweeter to the taste. David prays for strength from God to discern these delicacies, and resist buying into them.

For those who are able to resist the temptations of the tongue, David also addresses the temptations of the heart. Those who remain silent must also examine their thoughts and attitudes. Do they remain godly? When we do not get our way on the committee, or our plans and policy ideas are not followed, Christians must also resist brooding on the negative thoughts which our flesh conjures up. Paul's words should come to mind: "For our struggle is not against flesh and blood, but against the rulers, against the powers, against the world forces of this darkness, against the spiritual forces of wickedness in the heavenly places" (Eph. 6:12).

Psalm 141 continues this way:

> Let the righteous smite me in kindness and reprove me;
> it is oil upon the head;
> do not let my head refuse it. (v. 5)

In praying against temptation, and in enlisting God's help with an issue, the input of other Christians should be welcomed. God has made each Christian a member of the church, a part of the Body of Christ. Christians should not act as lone-ranger warriors or crusaders. Christians should expect, and desire, other Christians to come to them and confront them about issues in their lives. They should anticipate disagreements with brothers and sisters, and see them as important opportunities to improve their ideas (Prov. 27:17). But often disunity arises between Christians today when they seem to be astounded that other Christians would disagree with them, and then openly state so. Yet David shows us in this verse that it is important to pray that the righteous confront us on issues where we have differences.

In my own life, my closest friend in the Lord told me this past year that he believed my whole emphasis in ministry, and how I was spending my time, was unbalanced and unbiblical. In his eyes, writing and speaking at conferences could not be appropriate since it did not involve building long-term relationships with others, or leading others to Christ. Yet I believed God was leading me in this way, and was opening up many opportunities. My friend's comments hurt and worried me because he knows me very well. It scared me that I might have been deceived.

Proverbs 27:6 states: "Faithful are the wounds of a friend, but deceitful are the kisses of an enemy." (See also Eccl. 7:5.) Even though we disagreed, I benefited greatly from his raising this issue. We remain faithful friends. I was forced to think through why I spent my time the way I did. It forced me to struggle with how I came to know God's will for my life. It drove me back to God in a deeper way, because I was so afraid I might have deceived myself over what I thought God wanted me to do for him. After David was rebuked, he continued to pray against the deeds of the wicked. His goals did not change, and neither did mine.

Christians should have the privilege of having other Christians involved in their lives, helping them to focus more clearly on God's will for their lives. Christians need others who know them intimately, and are willing to advise or confront them when needed (Col. 1:28). The New Testament paints a picture of intimate fellowship between believers. Part of the role of the Body of Christ is to provide direction for Christians. If the plans and goals we pray for are not coming to fruition, the problem may be that others do not know us well enough to give advice on those plans. Christians should welcome the opportunity to have others love us enough to disagree with us, and constructively work on ways to improve our plans to make a difference.

Their judges are thrown down by the sides of the rock,
And they hear my words, for they are pleasant.

As when one plows and breaks open the earth,
Our bones have been scattered at the mouth of Sheol. (Ps. 141:6-7)

David now turns to the future. With his prayer against their wickedness, he has confidence that the wicked will be exposed and his words will be vindicated. Verse 7 is unclear, but carries the image of the sufferings David endured (scattering the bones). But rather than being defeated, the imagery of plowing brings to mind the death which allows a seed to grow and eventually be harvested. "Obscure as the language of this verse is, it carries the previous thought forward to its climax, reinforcing the resolve to strike no bargains with evil, by looking ahead to the time when such a stand will prove its point and win its following."[2]

The present situation may not give the appearance that many things are going God's way. Fewer may agree with Christian perspectives on issues, and even fewer abide by those perspectives. But Christians must have an eternal perspective. Eventually everyone will have to acknowledge that God exists, and his ways are right. But even before that, his way may be vindicated. Plans opposed to God will be destructive and ineffective. As other perspectives are tried and fail, people may be open to hearing God's perspective. Then God's words will be seen as pleasant (v. 6). This word literally means sweet or mild, and contrasts with the artificial "delicacies" of the world (v. 4).[3] Christians should remain hopeful, not in short-term results, but in the knowledge that God has won the ultimate victory, and at some point will be vindicated.

For my eyes are toward You, O God, the Lord;
In You I take refuge; do not leave me defenseless.
Keep me from the jaws of the trap which they have set for me,
And from the snares of those who do iniquity.
Let the wicked fall into their own nets,
While I pass by safely. (vv. 8-10)

David reminds us that his confidence is in God. He relies on God to get him through this situation, not his craftiness or weapons or good fortune. He knows that God is the one who will protect him from his enemies.

In the same way, Christians seeking to make a difference in the world

2. Derek Kidner, *Psalms 73–150: A Commentary on Books III-V of the Psalms* (London: Inter-Varsity Press, 1975), p. 472.
3. C. H. Spurgeon, *The Treasury of David* (New York: Association Press, 1913), 6:319.

need to first turn to God. They need to personally rely on him, not their intellect or education or financial means. When under attack, our refuge must be in him, not ourselves or our organizations or argumentativeness. At the same time, Christians should be alert to the craftiness of those who oppose God's ways. They are laying snares, and would like to see those who oppose them fall into their traps. These traps are often temptations to take the easy way out of the conflict, leading one commentary to view this psalm as "A prayer against insincerity and compromise, and a plea for survival under the savage attacks which such an attitude has invited."[4] If we do sometimes fall into one of these traps, we need to climb out on the shoulders of Christ, trusting in him to carry us through.

David concludes by recalling once more that God will take care of him. The final outcome is already determined: the very traps laid to capture him will ensnare the wicked who laid them, not David. He will pass safely by, confident in the Lord.

Christians should similarly be confident in the Lord as we seek to make an impact. We can take all sorts of risks in speaking out on difficult and controversial issues. We can hold to unpopular opinions. We can resist the temptations to buy into the dainty morsels that look so nice, but ultimately are unsatisfying. We can take these risks because we know we are safe. We are safe in the arms of the Lord who loves us and protects us. Christians can only make a difference if they start in the arms of the Lord. Time needs to be spent in prayer before stepping into the fray. But into the fray we must go. We can do so with confidence only if we have first turned to the Lord for the needed strength and direction.

So, let us turn to the Lord. Let us confess where we have previously gone astray, where we have embraced the delicacies of the comfortable life. Let us accept the encouragement and rebuke of our friends in the Lord. And let us remember that God is God. He has defeated the Evil One. He will take care of us. He is in control. And we have the opportunity to make a difference wherever we can shine his light on the world around us.

The Horizontal Dimension

Having turned vertically to the Lord in prayer to find security and confidence, Christians also have the power of prayer to make a difference horizontally: within the world. The greatest command is to love our Lord, but inseparable

4. Kidner, *Psalms 73–150*, p. 470.

from that is the command to love our neighbors (Matt. 22:37-40). Everything that Christians do should flow from their relationship with God. They should aim to be faithful to God, to bring glory to him, *and* to serve others. However, there is sometimes confusion over how prayer serves others. We question what the horizontal dimension of our prayer life looks like, and what we can expect to see through it.

There is much current interest within health care in prayer. More and more books are being written on the topic; news magazines have addressed the issue. From a Christian perspective, not all of this is positive.[5] One problem with this trend stems from what different people mean by prayer. For example, in *Prayer Works,* Rosemary Guiley views prayer as a vibrating inner connection with the divine. From this stems a view of prayer as control over esoteric powers. Guiley cites with approval the founder of the Unity School of Christianity: "Then it flashed upon me that I might talk to the life in every part of my body and have it do just what I wanted. I began to teach my body and got marvelous results. . . . I told the life in my abdomen that it was no longer infested with ignorant ideas of disease, put there by myself and by doctors, but that it was all a thrill with the sweet, pure, wholesome energy of God."[6]

Larry Dossey, M.D., author of the best-selling *Healing Words* and *Be Careful What You Pray For . . . You Just Might Get It,* sees prayer as a type of language.[7] He uses the term *prayerfulness* to express a general attitude of leaving things in the hands of a universal consciousness.[8] A prominent researcher in the field of prayer and healing calls prayer "distance healing" and defines it "as any purely mental effort undertaken by one person with the intention of improving physical or emotional well-being in another."[9] Others define prayer as a way to send impersonal healing energy, leading

---

5. For a more complete discussion of these issues see Dónal P. O'Mathúna, "Prayer Research: What Are We Measuring?" *Journal of Christian Nursing* 16, no. 3 (Summer 1999): 17-21.

6. Myrtle Fillmore, cited in Rosemary Ellen Guiley, *Prayer Works: True Stories of Answered Prayer* (Unity Village, Mo.: Unity Books, 1998), p. 12.

7. Larry Dossey, *Healing Words: The Power of Prayer and the Practice of Medicine* (New York: HarperSanFrancisco, 1993); *Prayer Is Good Medicine: How to Reap the Healing Benefits of Prayer* (New York: HarperSanFrancisco, 1996); *Be Careful What You Pray For . . . You Just Might Get It: What We Can Do About the Unintentional Effects of Our Thoughts, Prayers and Wishes* (New York: HarperSanFrancisco, 1997).

8. Dossey, *Healing Words,* pp. 5-8, 23-24.

9. Elisabeth Targ, "Evaluating Distant Healing: A Research Review," *Alternative Therapies in Health & Medicine* 3, no. 6 (November 1997): 74.

them to view prayer as the same as sorcery, shamanism, psychic healing, and telepathy.[10]

To Dossey's credit, he does make it clear that when he discusses prayer, he is talking about something very different from Christian prayer. He states that his view of prayer is "far different" from the "old biblically-based views of prayer," where people communicate with a personal God who is distinct and separate from humans.[11] According to Dossey, biblical prayer arises from a worldview that "is now antiquated and incomplete" and constitutes a "uniquely 'pathological mythology.'"[12] In contrast, many of the other authors claim their view of prayer is compatible with the Christian view. For example, the foreword to Guiley's book claims: "You can be a Christian or a Hindu, a Moslem or a Jew. Even an atheist can pray, for prayer does not depend upon belief, although belief might be the reason we sit or kneel or fall prostrate to the floor. . . . Prayer is tuning to a higher vibration until the divine connection is made."[13]

Christian prayer can only be seen as a humble request to the all-knowing, all-powerful God to bring about what he knows is best in a particular situation (Matt. 6:25-34). Prayer is not just a state of mind, although it certainly should impact one's state of mind (Phil. 4:6; 1 Thess. 5:17-18). Prayer is not just an energy which, once emitted, takes on a life of its own with predictable outcomes. This predictable view of prayer is intrinsic to doing research on the effects of healing prayer. While Christians are instructed to ask for specific outcomes, they must always acknowledge that specific requests will be granted only "if the Lord wills" (James 4:13-16; 1 John 5:14).

Christians seeking to make a difference in our world must first be discerning about what people are calling prayer. At the same time, people's interest in any form of prayer is an opportunity to engage in a dialogue about their views of prayer. Christians should prepare themselves for those opportunities by understanding their culture and what is viewed as prayer. Paul revealed his knowledge of the religious beliefs and practices of his day in Acts 17. Christians should seek out opportunities to engage people in these discussions, not be fearful of other views. Paul again is an example here, calling on us to pray for the words that will touch others' hearts and spirits:

---

10. Marilyn Schlitz and William Braud, "Distant Intentionality and Healing: Assessing the Evidence," *Alternative Therapies in Health & Medicine* 3, no. 6 (November 1997): 62-73; Dossey, *Be Careful*, pp. 11-13.

11. Dossey, *Healing Words*, pp. 6-7.

12. Dossey, *Healing Words*, p. 7.

13. Michael A. Maday, foreword in Guiley, *Prayer Works*, p. x.

Devote yourselves to prayer, keeping alert in it with an attitude of thanksgiving; praying at the same time for us as well, that God may open up to us a door for the word, so that we may speak forth the mystery of Christ, for which I have also been imprisoned; in order that I may make it clear in the way I ought to speak. Conduct yourselves with wisdom toward outsiders, making the most of the opportunity. Let your speech always be with grace, seasoned, as it were, with salt, so that you may know how you should respond to each person. (Col. 4:2-6)

The goal of these discussions, and focus of these prayers, should be to bring the ultimate healing power of God to bear in a person's life. The first thing that needs repair is a person's relationship with Jesus Christ. Jesus said that he came so that people might have life, and might have life abundantly (John 10:10). This only comes through each person accepting the sacrifice of Jesus Christ as payment for his or her sins (John 1:12-13). As Christians pray for others, they must keep in mind the need for this fundamental healing. Physical or emotional healing is secondary until spiritual healing has occurred. Additionally, Christians should not expect those who do not have a restored relationship with Christ to live as if they did.

However, Christians should still be praying for physical and emotional healing. There is ample reason to believe that God continues to heal people today, though probably not as often as some would like us to believe. James leaves us a very clear passage on prayer for healing, from which we can distil some helpful general guidelines.[14]

Is anyone among you suffering? Let him pray. Is anyone cheerful? Let him sing praises. Is anyone among you sick? Let him call for the elders of the church, and let them pray over him, anointing him with oil in the name of the Lord; and the prayer offered in faith will restore the one who is sick, and the Lord will raise him up, and if he has committed sins, they will be forgiven him. Therefore, confess your sins to one another, and pray for one another, so that you may be healed. The effective prayer of a righteous man can accomplish much. (James 5:13-16)

First, Christians who are suffering are instructed to pray. This should be the Christian response to negative circumstances. This prayer is also described as a corporate activity. This assumes a level of involvement in one another's lives that allows Christians to know who is sick and suffering. From this should stem the freedom to share these requests with one another.

14. A very helpful and concise pamphlet on this subject is Douglas Connelly, *How Can I Pray When I'm Sick?* (Downers Grove, Ill.: InterVarsity, 1999).

Second, the sick person is to call the elders for anointing. There is still a place for anointing of the sick. The significance of the oil is twofold. Oil had important symbolic value. The disciples who were sent out by Jesus anointed the sick when they healed them (Mark 6:13). As in the Old Testament, oil was closely associated with the work of God. "Consequently, oil was a powerful reminder to the church that God was able to heal and that his healing powers were already being made manifest."[15] At the same time, oil was used in biblical times for its medicinal purposes. From this, and other passages, we can affirm the use of appropriate medications by those who are sick. So, as long as they are part of God's good creation, and not spiritually entangled, medical treatments can be seen as natural aspects of God's provision for healing.[16] There is nothing to suggest that prayer for healing should be the only way to deal with an illness.

Third, James brings up the whole area of confession. He makes it clear, however, that it is only *if* a person has sinned that confession when sick is needed. In his thorough study of New Testament healing, John Christopher Thomas shows that in those cases where confession is part of healing, the person knew what his or her sin was.[17] Healing can be from God, but so can suffering. God promises to discipline those whom he loves (Heb. 12:4-13). This may include sending an illness to get someone's attention. In those cases, however, the person will know what he or she needs to confess. At the same time, Jesus makes it clear that all sickness is not the result of sin. In Luke 13 he makes it clear that the people killed by Herod or the falling tower in Siloam were not worse sinners than those who escaped. In John 9 Jesus is also clear that the man was not born blind because of his sin or that of his parents. But sometimes, God may use an illness to get our attention on an issue. In those cases, repentance and confession will lead to healing.

Finally, James goes on in verses 17-18 of chapter 5 to remind us of the example of Elijah and the way his prayer led to the drought and to the rain starting again later. What was it that made Elijah's prayer so effective? The actual accounts show that Elijah's close relationship with God led him to know what to pray for (1 Kings 17–18). Elijah did not think up this "rain test" as a way to research God's reality. God came to him and told him what he would do, and what Elijah should tell the people. In the same way, we have God's

15. John Christopher Thomas, *The Devil, Disease and Deliverance: Origins of Illness in New Testament Thought* (Sheffield: Sheffield Academic Press, 1998), p. 28.
16. Dónal P. O'Mathúna, "Emerging Alternative Therapies," in *The Changing Face of Health Care: A Christian Appraisal,* ed. John F. Kilner, Robert D. Orr, and Judith Allen Shelly (Grand Rapids: Eerdmans, 1998), pp. 258-79.
17. Thomas, *The Devil, Disease and Deliverance.*

guidance on certain things we know are true. We can be confident that he will answer those prayers.

But we must also acknowledge that we often do not know if it is God's will to heal everyone. Job was a righteous man (Job 1:1) but God allowed him to suffer excruciating physical illness (Job 1:7-8), although he was eventually healed. Timothy appears to have been sickly (1 Tim. 5:23). Epaphroditus was even made sick by his work in the ministry (Phil. 2:25-30). Paul had a thorn in the flesh, which is usually believed to have been some physical illness. He prayed against it, asking God to remove it (2 Cor. 12:7-10). Yet it was not removed. As Paul realized God was not going to heal him, he reflected on how he could deal with his less than perfect body:

> And because of the surpassing greatness of the revelations, for this reason, to keep me from exalting myself, there was given me a thorn in the flesh, a messenger of Satan to buffet me — to keep me from exalting myself! Concerning this I entreated the Lord three times that it might depart from me. And He has said to me, "My grace is sufficient for you, for power is perfected in weakness." Most gladly, therefore, I will rather boast about my weaknesses, that the power of Christ may dwell in me. Therefore I am well content with weaknesses, with insults, with distresses, with persecutions, with difficulties, for Christ's sake; for when I am weak, then I am strong.

In conclusion, we should turn to God in the midst of the situations we find ourselves within. We can have confidence that he is there, waiting for us with open arms. However, he does not give us a guarantee that our prayers will be answered the way we want. Whether we would like to see a sickness healed, a policy passed, or a vote go a particular way, we should seek the Lord's input through prayer. We can lay our burdens at his feet. But we should do so humbly, knowing that God will bring about what is best. That may not be in our lifetime, but ultimately God's will shall be done on earth. It is our responsibility to pray for this, and take those steps of action God lays in front of us. We are to be faithful servants of the Lord, not messiahs. The Messiah has come once, and will return on the day of ultimate victory.

PART II

EDUCATION AND THE MEDIA

The New Medicine and the Education of the Christian Mind

Nigel M. de S. Cameron, Ph.D.

The gathering pace of fundamental cultural change is pitching us ever nearer to the consistently post-Christian society. This change represents a radical shift in the belief- and value-systems of our civilization. And while there are complex dimensions to cultures and their interconnections, "Western" culture — this increasingly incoherent amalgam of classical, Judeo-Christian, and post-Christian components — is far and away the dominant force in the emerging global society. At the heart of the new pattern of understanding, in which we are regrouping around post-Christian assumptions and as the defaults are reset, lies the question of bioethics. It is as significant as that.[1]

Yet among all the changes taking place in the culture, and despite the public and religious importance of the issue of abortion, we know that bioethics itself is a Cinderella; even in our churches, which have a compelling interest in the question of human being, once we get beyond abortion, bioethics and its myriad questions come low on any list of priority concerns.

The explanation lies partly in the fixation we have with effects, inversely and obtusely proportioned to our interest in causes. If it is an exaggeration to suggest that the social-cultural agenda of the conservative church consists of a shower of epiphenomena, it is a pardonable one. The challenge to address systemic questions, matters of disease rather than merely its symptoms, is hard to underscore too much. The cultural incompetence of the church of

---

1. The broad context of current developments in bioethics is explored in my book *The New Medicine: Life and Death after Hippocrates* (Wheaton, Ill.: Crossway, 1992).

our day lies partly here, in its absorption with problems to the exclusion of the problem. And the problem, in bioethics as elsewhere, is the need to articulate a Christian worldview as the starting-point of cultural engagement. That in turn opens our eyes to the central educational challenge we face.

The abortion controversy offers an illuminating example of our problem. On the one hand it has galvanized Christian opinion, and has drawn many individuals into bioethics as well as catalyzed great numbers of Christians into some awareness of the shifts taking place in the Judeo-Christian values of the culture. Yet at the same time, this most dramatic symptom of our malaise has been seen as an end in itself, as if abortion is what is wrong with the culture. It has not been seen, as it should be, as the most striking and widespread example of the tragic folly that results from the abandonment of the Hippocratic vision for medicine, which was long sustained by the Christian moral underpinnings of the West. This essential misunderstanding of the significance of the question of abortion has had major practical implications, not least in the matter of funding. If, let us say, one-tenth of the resources which have been devoted to the abortion issue since *Roe* had been tithed for the development of research into the future of bioethics, our capacity to address the coming tidal wave of new questions (from nanotechnology to cryopreservation) would have been strengthened immeasurably. This is not to say that we should have devoted fewer resources to abortion: they have been little enough. Yet our thinking about resources has lacked strategic focus. The recent example of the statement on stem-cell research in which this writer and other contributors to this book were involved offers an example of bricks without straw: it is a controversy in which we find ourselves pitted against the multi-billion-dollar appropriations of the National Institutes of Health.

Yet the strategic issue goes deeper still. The root of any culture, ancient or modern, lies in its conception of what it means to be human; its understanding of human identity offers the major premise to every particular of its cultural life. The steady assumption of the Western tradition that to have membership in *Homo sapiens* is to bear the *imago Dei*, an assumption that has given rise over time to so many of the advantages and benisons of our culture, is undergoing radical reshaping in the laboratory. This first principle of our tradition is being rewritten. The entire bioethics enterprise is focused at just this point: the redefining of the rules of engagement for human being, the practical ethical structures that determine how we should treat each other and ourselves, and that flow ineradicably from assumptions as to who we are.

A classic instance of this process can be found in the Warnock Report, the British government's recommendations in the early 1980s concerning in vitro fertilization and related matters.[2] In response to many submissions to the committee focusing on the central question of the identity of the human embryo, the report's writers make a conscious and overt decision to avoid addressing the question of the nature of the embryo at all. They state that they will instead proceed immediately to the deliberative question of how to treat the human embryo. The issue of course is particularly pressing in the case of the embryo, since to establish that the embryo is "one of us" is immediately to set the debate in a context in which the protection of this smallest member of *Homo sapiens* is paramount. This sidestepping of the question of identity draws striking attention to the central problem of contemporary bioethics. Sidestepping the question, sometimes done deftly, sometimes less so, is typical. Next the tendency is to "address" it with a raft of procedural responses that claim adequacy of their own and yet in fact reveal the outlines of some other, post-Christian, understanding of human nature.

The Warnock Report, and subsequent handlings of the debate, illustrate the gravity of the situation we face — a situation especially grave in light of such limited interest and understanding on the part of the Christian church. Further, we clearly see the need for education, both of our own committed constituencies, and in the public square, because the discussion of bioethics is very complicated.

Let us now look at some practical educational possibilities. The state of our Christian churches, colleges, seminaries, and other institutions reveals the scale of the need and corresponding opportunity. With very few exceptions, they are making little or no effort to educate their students, members, constituents, readers, and listeners in the matter which, if we are correct, is where the old culture and the new have begun to do battle to define the future of humankind.[3]

1. Christian Schools

Christian colleges and universities are the place to begin. They represent the deposit of faith of generations of Christians who have believed in the importance of education and the necessity of engaging the great questions of the day. Their birthright is to be "worldview" institutions: they speak generally of

2. See *Embryos and Ethics: The Warnock Report in Debate*, ed. Nigel M. de S. Cameron (Edinburgh: Rutherford House, 1987).

3. Publishing is a further area. *Ethics and Medicine* remains the sole journal that addresses bioethics from the perspective of a biblically informed Christian faith. (Details may be obtained from The Center for Bioethics and Human Dignity.)

the "integration" of faith and learning. While this offers an ambiguous locution (it seems to suggest that the two are not in themselves coherent; it is of course rather a methodological reflection on the need to re-integrate the two in the post-Enlightenment world), their entire mission is to develop world-view Christians.

The extent to which this is accomplished is unclear. Most Christian schools certainly could enhance their effectiveness, especially in relation to their pre-professional majors, pre-medicine in particular.

One exception is Trinity International University in Deerfield, Illinois, on whose campus is the Center for Bioethics and Human Dignity. During the 1990s, Trinity established a series of programs in bioethics, including an undergraduate minor (the only such program in North America, as far as is known). Graduate programs include seminary master of arts and master of divinity emphases as well as a doctor of ministry track in bioethics for chaplaincy. Within Trinity Graduate School, and as a joint degree at Trinity Law School in Santa Ana, California, there is also a specialist master of arts in bioethics. These are apparently the only such programs in evangelical schools worldwide.

It is a curious fact, and a haunting comment on the depth of our problem, that most religious schools offering pre-med programs have no bioethics requirement whatever; their pre-med training is understood essentially as a chemistry or physics sequence intended to help students get into medical school. The lack of imagination that has given rise to this situation is hard to explain, since no institution is more committed in principle, or prepared in practice, to articulate the Christian worldview than a Christian college.

Seminaries have a special challenge, since every pastor every week faces issues of bioethics. Infertile couples, elderly hospital patients and their relatives — even in routine situations, the bioethics agenda is pressing. Yet pastoral training offers little or no preparation for these uniquely difficult challenges. Such a lack reflects several factors. They include the general evangelical unease with ethics, which as a whole is generally relegated to a single course in the required master of divinity curriculum (Roman Catholic institutions, with their long tradition of moral philosophy, are more effective here). Also, in more traditional seminaries biblical languages and basic Bible teaching dominate the curriculum (and in schools that have revised the traditional curriculum, counseling and management issues have become the focus). There also is a failure, often on the part of faculty whose pastoral experience did not encompass such things, to understand the pervasive importance of these new questions; and a general disinclination to engage in the kind of radical restructuring of the curriculum that would give appropriate place to the vital importance of preparing pastors to help their congregations engage the culture within the framework of the Christian worldview.

Yet what of the curriculum? The graduate program at Trinity was devised in response to study of curricula offered at a dozen major schools with bioethics programs, often found in philosophy departments. Plainly, a Christian bioethics program will nest in theology, especially systematic theology with its philosophical as well as biblical foundations. It will have its prime focus on method, addressing the nature of the human person in light of every relevant discipline. It will cover the history and nature of bioethics, seeking to tie this neologism of a discipline to its forebears in the older "medical ethics" and moral philosophy, as well as to locate its birth in the 1960s and 1970s in the context of the general revolt against the values of the Western tradition. It will focus professionally (and this is one point at which the Trinity programs have far to go). The revival of the professional idea is central to the Christian stake in contemporary bioethics, and is a powerful point of contact with some of the most positive concerns in contemporary culture. Bioethics as a philosophical and inter-disciplinary field represents the failure of medicine to retain a moral vision. While more than physicians and nurses should be involved in bioethics, the revival of the professional idea along Hippocratic lines would set the discussion back in its proper context.

In institutional terms, Christian higher education has been much too dependent on large blocks of Bible and religion in its undergraduate curriculum. By extension, where graduate programs have developed in non-religious fields there has been pressure to add "Bible and religion" requirements to ensure the orthodoxy of the program. Ironically, this can prove entirely counterproductive; it offers a seeming shield for institutional integrity that can readily free the remainder of the curriculum from primary responsibility for "integrative" (or worldview) teaching. While the curriculum may be well-served by assigning responsibility for Bible and religion to some separate courses, the basic worldview function of the program must always be borne by the disciplinary courses. By the same token, the task of the Bible and religion instructors should be, as it were, "pre-worldview"; that is, carefully and intentionally articulated with disciplinary instruction. The decoupling of the two is, of course, the weakest point of Christian higher education; and the opportunity to enhance incrementally its effectiveness in the preparation of worldview Christians may be directly proportionate to the effectiveness of the curricular "couple" which must radically affect all aspects of both kinds of courses. A congruent recognition of the "pre-worldview" character of all seminary instruction would impart a dynamic quality to what can all too easily become static, content-focused preparation, and give worldview torque to pastoral preparation for mindset leadership in the twenty-first-century church.

2. Professional Networks

Christian professional networks have in various ways begun to take up the challenge of articulating and inculcating the distinctives of the Christian worldview, and especially the implications — for physicians, nurses, attorneys, and others — of the development of bioethics. These networks, which generally began as fellowships for Christians working in the different fields, and then developed evangelistic and other goals, now face a daunting challenge. Because they are directly involved in some of the largest changes under way in our culture, they need to give countercultural leadership in the post-Christian era.

The professions as such are conservative bodies that focus the marriage of value and technique that has formed their professional identity and whose moral vision for the exercise of skills has led to their possessing a high order of both public and private trust. Yet Christians within the professions find themselves seeking to hold or call back their colleagues to standards that were once widely embraced in the culture. The questions of bioethics will increasingly prove central to the definition of medicine and the related professions. The task facing Christians is to rise to the challenge, and to use their networks to ensure serious understanding of the bioethics agenda. No longer are these matters peripheral (if ever they were) or even secondary (which many would still see them to be). They hold center stage in the culture, and therefore should be at the forefront of attention for Christians within the professions.

3. The Churches

Evangelical churches themselves are in a curious position. On the one hand, there is enormous pressure on them to fulfill all kinds of roles that actually threaten their identity as the church of Jesus Christ. Every pastor in the land is deluged with requests that he or she promote activities and messages and products from agencies good, bad, and irrelevant. It is ironic that in resisting the pressure to focus on social-cultural questions — a generally healthy response that has been seasoned by the fundamentalist tradition of cultural denial and that recognizes the widespread failure of the old "social gospel" movement that the fundamentalists decried — conservative churches have contributed to the secularizing of the culture by their reluctance or simple in-capacity to engage their members in "worldview" Christian living. That is to say, they have determined to focus on the Christian religion in such a manner as has in effect denied one of its central tenets. Christians have not been en-couraged to see their (largely "secular") vocations as God-given; they have been taught the Bible as if its only concern were the performance of religious activities; they have been denied any serious understanding of the fact that God remains the Creator and that Jesus Christ told his followers to be "in" the world, even as he told them not to be "of" it.

This is of course a broader question than one just affecting bioethics, but it sets the context for medicine and bioethics as for other questions. The church has a prime responsibility to prepare its people to live "in" the world according to principles that come from God. It is remarkable, for instance, that so many Christians seeking help in having a child fail to grasp the moral significance, for example, of reproductive technology, and find themselves led through referrals into using in vitro or surrogacy or some other questionable benefit of the new technology — with no context for their decisions set in Christian education within the local church. It is hard to see how any church could avoid addressing the bioethics agenda in Sunday school and pulpit teaching, youth ministry, wedding preparation, young marrieds' groups — indeed, throughout its educa-tional task. On the other hand, if this does not happen it reflects sharply on the pastor's and church leaders' education, which in so many of our seminaries is disconnected from the radical cultural context in which they are being called to minister. If the seminary student is prepared to be the interpreter of the culture, if a key function of his or her role is seen as that of developing a Christian worldview in the mind of the fellowship, if a central question addressed to would-be pastors is how well they have mastered this task — our church would be different, and so would our society. By expecting Christians to engage cul-ture rather than disengage from it, we would free ourselves to be "salt" and "leaven" and cease to aid the process of secularization that comes from evacuat-ing ourselves from the culture in a confused attempt to keep ourselves pure (and, of course, to enable us to focus more on "religious" activities).

The educational task facing the church is therefore as follows. We need to prepare this generation for the redefinition of our humanity, and to teach believers how to live out the vision of human dignity made in God's image in a bioethics culture where such a vision is being supplanted with other and as yet unresolved alternatives. The significance of this undertaking as we move into what many expect will be a culture in which euthanasia has been em-braced as routinely as abortion, and in which traditional childbearing within marriage may come to be the exception, is potentially devastating.

4. Bioethics Centers

If we are looking to leverage cultural influence, we need to start centers, mini-institutions of thought that are often called "think tanks." If a Bible text were sought for the establishment of centers, it might be "a little leaven leavens the whole lump." Centers are yeast for our culture: in skilled hands, they can allow tiny proportions of input to result in huge outputs. The Center for Bioethics and Human Dignity in Illinois, and the Centre for Bioethics and Public Policy in London, are two striking examples of projects that although modestly funded have succeeded in focusing major discussions during the rapidly advancing bioethics agenda of the 1990s.[4]

Centers, or institutes, or think tanks, have begun to wield disproportionate influence on many fronts during this time of cultural redefinition and shift. But it is specially true in bioethics, which is the quintessentially postmodern discipline. In this field centers and journals and conferences are the parallel to the laboratories and great libraries and large faculties of the more established disciplines. Form follows function here; bioethics is distinctly postmodern in both. The structure of bioethics reflects its character as a discipline on the move, an exercise of intellectual revolutionaries who have taken a leading role in the reshaping of the West in its turbulent, unconstrained, post-Christian commitment to health and technology.

The development of the Internet, the ease of small publishing, the flexibility of work patterns, the globalization of our agenda — all these and other features of our culture at the start of the twenty-first century are gifts to members of a relatively small, internationally strong, countercultural movement that seeks to draw on the stability and coherence of our Judeo-Christian and Hippocratic traditions as the context in which to address the unfolding bioethics agenda. We seek also to bring our perspectives to bear persuasively and pervasively across the international frontiers of the conversation. We need a major investment in the seeding of non-traditional institutions — with their relatively low cost and potentially high profile (once established in the Rolodexes of the press), capacity to collaborate across national boundaries and pursue debates around the globe, and ability to use the Internet for building communities and all means of communication (they should readily be able to match, if not surpass, the Web presence of their rivals). Some participants in this movement may be connected with traditional institutions or have links with other non-profits and networks; others will be self-standing.

---

4. A new project that addresses a vital aspect of the debate should be noted: The Center for Bioethics in the Church (www.thecbc.org).

They can draw on the best in Christian thinking, both on the issues and on how to communicate with each other and in the public square.

*   *   *

As we move into the third millennium, let us gird up our countercultural loins and engage these great questions that will set the parameters of the culture's new vision of what it means to be human. Let us determine to inform the church of Jesus Christ, so that believers might understand the significance of the bioethics agenda, learn how to face these questions for themselves, and speak to their generation in both prophecy and translation. Let us resolve to let loose the people of God to uphold the dignity of *Homo sapiens,* as the creature of God's image. For at the heart of the contemporary crisis in bioethics we face nothing more nor less than a rerun of the Enlightenment belief in humankind as the measure of all things. And of course that philosophy is doomed to fail, again. It is scarcely irrelevant that the twentieth century — ending as it is in this great effort at post-Christian reconstruction of human identity in the context of medicine and the bio-sciences — will haunt the history of the world as the home of the two great anti-Christian systems that elevated the human spirit at the expense of its subjection to God, communism and national socialism.

"Glory to man in the highest,/for man is the master of things."

Thus wrote A. C. Swinburne, Victorian neo-pagan and prophet of the twentieth century. Only in retrospect, at century's end, do we gain something of the full tragic significance of that early sampling of post-Christian bravado. If the twenty-first is not going to replicate that impious vision on its own Huxleyian terms, the church of Jesus Christ must be informed and it must speak soft, loud, in season and out of season, the words *imago Dei.*

Strategies for Sex Education

Mary B. Adam, M.D.

In the United States, about 12 million new cases of sexually transmitted diseases (STDs) occur annually, with 3 million cases in teenagers. Estimates of the annual direct and indirect costs of selected major STDs are approximately $10 billion and if HIV infections are included, costs rise to about $17 billion. This cost is shared among all Americans through higher healthcare costs and higher taxes. STDs disproportionately affect women and adolescents. Women are more vulnerable to STDs because they are biologically more susceptible to certain diseases than men and they are more likely to have asymptomatic infections that often result in delays in diagnosis and treatment. From 1973-1992 more than 150,000 women died of causes associated with STDs and their complications. Reported rates of curable STDs are several times higher in the United States than in other developed countries. Adolescents have a greater risk of STDs than adults for a number of reasons that include multiple sexual partners, having sexual partners who are at higher risk of having STDs, and being more likely to engage in intercourse without a condom. By the twelfth grade 27 percent of high school students have had four or more sexual partners. If one takes into account that not all teens are sexually active, the actual risk for acquiring an STD among sexually experienced teenagers may be significantly higher than the data suggests.[1]

The magnitude of the problem internationally is best exemplified by looking at the HIV epidemic. In some sub-Saharan African cities the preva-

---

1. Institute of Medicine, *The Hidden Epidemic: Confronting Sexually Transmitted Diseases* (Washington, D.C.: National Academy Press, 1997), pp. 1, 29, 36, 49, 103.

lence of HIV infection in pregnant women is as high as 33 percent.[2] All this leads one to the conclusion that STDs are an epidemic of tremendous consequence both in the United States and abroad.

Sex education has been credited as having a fundamental role in reducing STDs and adolescent pregnancies. In 1986, then Surgeon General C. Everett Koop called for sex education in the schools as an important facet in combating the AIDS epidemic. Sex education in the schools has also been seen as essential in responding to the epidemic of adolescent pregnancies. Currently, the Centers for Disease Control in Atlanta reports that over 90 percent of students have received some type of sex education.[3]

But what kind of sex education is needed? The debate over what type of sex education rages across the country from school boards to Congress. It is a minefield for all who venture into the area. The attitudes expressed by persons from various viewpoints are often vehement and emotional. At the root of this hostility are fundamental differences in how we, as individuals and as a society, understand human sexuality. These conflicts, both perceived and real, can be traced to differences in worldview.

While there are many kinds of sex education programs aimed at school-aged children, they can be divided into two camps based on their primary strategy. In one camp, the primary strategy is aimed at risk reduction. The other camp aims its primary strategy at risk avoidance. These differences in primary strategy reflect differences in worldview. A risk reduction strategy, one that would promote condoms and contraception, fits with a postmodern, feminist, or naturalist worldview. A risk avoidance strategy, which emphasizes sexual abstinence until marriage and then lifelong monogamy, reflects a Judeo-Christian perspective.

Nowhere has this collision of opposing approaches to sex education been more obvious than in the discussions surrounding the $250 million in federal funds dedicated to abstinence-only sex education, which Congress passed in 1996 as part of welfare reform. The law calls for teaching that a "mutually faithful, monogamous relationship in the context of marriage is the only appropriate setting for sexual intercourse."[4] A mutually faithful, monogamous relationship in the context of marriage is consistent with a Judeo-

---

2. P. Way, B. Schwartlander, and P. Piot, "The Global Epidemiology of HIV and AIDS," in *Sexually Transmitted Diseases,* ed. K. Holmes, P. A. Mardh, and P. F. Sparling et al. (New York: McGraw-Hill, 1999), pp. 77-94.

3. L. Kann, S. A. Kinchen, and B. I. Williams et al., "Youth risk behavior surveillance — United States, 1997," *MMWR CDC Surveill Summ.* 47 (1998): 1-89.

4. Personal Responsibility and Work Opportunity Act of 1996. P.L. 104-193, Title IX, Sec. 912. 1996.

Christian view of human sexuality. It calls for people to conform to an external standard and states that there is only one appropriate setting for sexual intercourse. Sex education, according to this view, would teach sexual abstinence until marriage and lifelong monogamy, or risk avoidance as the primary strategy. Risk avoidance programs would also disseminate information, teach refusal skills and decision making but these programs would tell people that they should choose lifelong monogamy as the only 100 percent effective choice, and that the only really "safe sex is saved sex," in other words, saved for marriage.

However, many people would disagree that marriage is the only appropriate setting for sexual intercourse. Those that consider lifelong monogamous marriage as abnormal, like postmodernists, feminists or, naturalists, would disagree with such an exclusive position and would consider such a view foolish, intolerant, and judgmental. Postmodernists and feminists categorically reject absolutist claims for truth or conduct and say that individuals must make a personal decision about their conduct based on their own internal standard of right and wrong. Naturalists see "right and wrong" as simply behaviors with a survival advantage and would make sexual choices based on what would promote their survival. Therefore those who hold these ideologies would promote those sex education programs that give information, allow people to examine their values, learn skills that would protect them from STDs, and become responsible sexually healthy adults. To be a sexually healthy adult would not require lifelong sexual monogamy. Therefore the primary educational strategy would be that of risk reduction or what is commonly called "safe sex." The main message would be "use a condom."

Even when teaching sexual abstinence it would be with an eye toward risk reduction as opposed to risk avoidance. Sexual abstinence could be presented as abstaining until you are ready as opposed to until you are married. Or it could be defined as mutual masturbation to orgasm but without penile vaginal intercourse. Former Surgeon General Joycelyn Elders, for example, was well known for promotion of mutual masturbation as an "abstinence" methodology. Many parents as well as those who consider themselves "abstinence only" promoters would call Elders' definition of abstinence, or mutual masturbation, a more unrealistic option than true abstinence, and say that it is playing with adolescent hormonal fire.

An excellent example of these conflicting ideologies with their corresponding primary educational strategies is found in an article from the July 3, 1999, edition of the *Tucson Citizen* entitled, "Condom dispensers, chastity programs at odds," which reads:

The state will push abstinence as Planned Parenthood sells contraceptives. While state lawmakers are pouring $3.5 million into promoting sexual abstinence to teen-agers, the local chapter of Planned Parenthood is starting a campaign that will place condom dispensers around Tucson. "It is not a good idea to send mixed messages, and the focus of our (state) campaign is sexual abstinence until marriage," said Brad Christenson, a spokesman for the Arizona Department of Health Services. Nevertheless, Planned Parenthood of Southern Arizona plans to spend $600,000 over the next three years on its new Protection Connection campaign that will include "Use Condom Sense" advertisements on Sun Tran benches and buses. Condom machines will be placed in locations youth frequent, such as movie theaters and social clubs. Condoms will cost 50 cents each. Dispensers will be brightly colored, in a symbolic reference to Lifesavers candies. Officials say that's because condoms save lives, prevent sexually transmitted diseases and unwanted pregnancies.[5]

In this article, sexual abstinence until marriage is pitted against the idea of safe sex, which translates to "have sex with the partners of your choice but use a condom." The fundamental clash here is not if one should be sexually active at all, but instead is over how many lifetime sexual partners one should be free to have. The conflict boils over into which STD prevention strategy should be taught to minors. The article goes on to state correctly that 27 percent of United States high school seniors have had four or more sexual partners. The implication is that compassion would require that these students be taught how to protect themselves. If you reject a Judeo-Christian worldview, you are left with no choice but a risk reduction strategy such as condoms. While postmodernists, feminists, or naturalists could tolerate lifelong sexual monogamy as a personal choice for those who would choose it, there is no philosophic justification for expecting people to make that choice. Risk avoidance is abandoned or at least relegated to the least helpful option, since no one is likely to choose it.

The "freedom" to have multiple sexual partners puts one at significant risk for STDs. Freedom always comes at a cost. The cost is paid by that individual who suffers the consequences of contracting an STD, a cost that ranges from mild inconvenience to death. In a "compassionate response" to that suffering, many organizations, such as Planned Parenthood in the above example, say "Reduce your risk. Use a condom." Yet the actual level of risk reduction for any given STD is never stated. This translates into a generic mantra,

---

5. S. Innes, "Condom dispensers, chastity programs at odds," *Tucson Citizen,* July 3, 1999.

"If you want to be safe use a condom" as if condoms were a foolproof method of protection. Unfortunately they are not.

The irony of this idea — that teaching adolescents how to protect themselves by using a condom is compassionate — is that it assumes people cannot and should not be trusted to tell the truth about their sexual history. People lie. You need to protect yourself. Or so say those whose views are rooted in self-interest and survival. Simplistic STD prevention messages result. Lydia Temoshok, Ph.D., has stated it well:

> HIV educators have continued to insist that people will only understand a simple message — use a condom every time. These educators think that it is better policy to tell people to use a condom with each partner, whether that partner is a spouse or a bar "pick up," than to advise people not to have sex at all with "casual" or anonymous partners. To justify this stance, and to negate the importance of testing and notification as prevention strategies, HIV educators insist that people lie about their past and present sexual lives: a husband or wife will deny an extramarital affair; the person you met through a shared interest group in your community will say they had an HIV test and that it was negative when in fact they never were tested; an HIV-infected person will not inform you of his/her positive status because of fear of rejection. Because you can't trust anyone, you should just use a condom every time with every partner.[6]

When philosophies that emphasize self-interest (naturalism's survival of the fittest) or individual rights (postmodernism or feminism) become the currency of human relationships, trust becomes bankrupt. When self-interest is the operational mode for human relationships, when "what you get," not "what you give," becomes the most important aspect of sexual relationships, then it is clear you can never trust your partner. When trust is destroyed, so is true intimacy. This leads one to question how compassionate a risk reduction strategy really is.

For that matter, so do the medical facts. The incurable nature of the viral STDs (Herpes, Human Papilloma Virus, and HIV) gives everyone pause when evaluating a risk reduction primary strategy like condoms. The medical facts about the efficacy of condoms in preventing transmission of HIV versus Chlamydia or Human Papilloma Virus (HPV) also give one pause. While condoms are about 90 percent effective in decreasing HIV

---

6. L. Temoshok, "Preventing the Transmission of the Human Immunodeficiency Virus," Feb. 5, 1998, 105th Cong., House Committee on Commerce, Subcommittee on Health and Environment, Serial 105-71, pp. 100-109.

transmission when correctly and consistently used, they have not been shown to reduce risk of Chlamydia (which causes increased rates of pelvic inflammatory disease, ectopic pregnancy, and infertility) or HPV infection in human trials (HPV causes more than 93 percent of all cervical cancer).[7] In the United States Chlamydia rates rose 250 percent over the ten-year period from 1986-1996.[8] Studies show that on college campuses 30 percent of women coeds are infected with HPV and 15 percent have the cancer-causing serotype.[9] According to a Centers for Disease Control study, the leading cause of STD-related death among women in the years 1973-1992 was cervical cancer (57 percent of deaths) followed by AIDS (27 percent of deaths).[10] In addition, while condoms are about 90 percent effective in preventing the transmission of HIV, some strains of HIV have been found to be exceedingly infectious. Recent reports document that one HIV-infected

7. E. J. Wilkinson, S. Malik, National Institutes of Health Consensus Development Conference statement on cervical cancer, April 1-3, 1996, *Journal of Women's Health* 7 (1998): 604-5; M. J. Rosenberg, A. J. Davidson, J. H. Chen, F. N. Judson, and J. M. Douglas, "Barrier contraceptives and sexually transmitted diseases in women: a comparison of female-dependent methods and condoms," *Am. J. Public Health* 82 (1992): 669-74; J. M. Zelin, A. J. Robinson, G. L. Ridgway, E. Allason-Jones, and P. Williams, "Chlamydial urethritis in heterosexual men attending a genitourinary medicine clinic: prevalence, symptoms, condom usage and partner change," *Int. J. STD. AIDS* 6 (1995): 27-30; J. M. Zenilman, C. S. Weisman, and A. M. Rompalo et al., "Condom use to prevent incident STDs: the validity of self-reported condom use," *Sex. Transm. Dis.* 22 (1995): 15-21; D. P. Orr, C. D. Langefeld, B. P. Katz, and V. A. Caine, "Behavioral intervention to increase condom use among high-risk female adolescents," *Journal of Pediatrics* 128 (1996): 288-95; S. C. Weller, "A meta-analysis of condom effectiveness in reducing sexually transmitted HIV," *Social Science & Medicine* 36 (1993): 1635-44; A. Saracco, M. Musicco, and A. Nicolosi et al., "Man-to-woman sexual transmission of HIV: longitudinal study of 343 steady partners of infected men," *J. Acquir. Immune. Defic. Syndr.* 6 (1993): 497-502; I. de Vincenzi, "A longitudinal study of human immunodeficiency virus transmission by heterosexual partners," European Study Group on Heterosexual Transmission of HIV, *N. Engl. J. Med.* 331 (1994): 341-46.

8. Division of STD Prevention, Sexually Transmitted Disease Surveillance 1996, U.S. Dept. of Health and Human Services, Public Health Service (Atlanta: Centers for Disease Control and Prevention, September 1997).

9. R. D. Burk, G. Y. Ho, L. Beardsley, M. Lempa, M. Peters, and R. Bierman, "Sexual behavior and partner characteristics are the predominant risk factors for genital human papillomavirus infection in young women," *Journal of Infectious Diseases* 174 (1996): 679-89.

10. S. H. Ebrahim, T. A. Peterman, and M. L. Kamb, "Mortality related to sexually transmitted diseases in women, U.S., 1973-1992" (Proceedings of the Eleventh Meeting of the International Society for STD Research, New Orleans, La., Aug. 27, 1995).

person passed HIV on to 13 of his 42 sexual partners and two of their infants, for an attack rate of over 30 percent.[11]

The battle over what the primary message of sex education should be is not surprising when one understands that the Judeo-Christian worldview no longer is the dominant view in this culture. Worldviews that elevate individual autonomy tend to dominate public policy. "Sexual abstinence until marriage" is an unusual message in a culture where sex sells everything from cars to vegetables, and movies like "American Pie" glorify casual sex and make fun of virginity. Yet the medical evidence also mirrors a fact so profound that the light of understanding is almost blinding. A lifelong mutually faithful monogamous sexual relationship is 100 percent effective in preventing the sexual transmission of disease. All other prevention methods are intrinsically limited. The logic of risk reduction makes eminent epidemiological sense, but when a physician is confronted with a weeping teenage patient who has primary herpes with open sores from her navel to her knees, risk reduction fails to provide comfort. It is not exactly what parents want for their children. The cost of a risk reduction approach in terms of medical sequela, human relationships, and expense of disease treatment leads one to question how compassionate this strategy really is. Is it really compassionate? Or is it a false panacea for those whose personal philosophy, whether articulated or not, gives them no better choice?

Is there common ground in this battle over primary strategy for sex education in the schools? Yes. And that common ground begins when one remembers the suffering of those individuals who have been infected with an STD.

It is the magnitude of those in need, suffering from emotional and physical pain caused by STDs, that returns people from various perspectives back to a common goal: that of eliminating STDs. It has driven the search for drugs to treat them and vaccines to prevent them. Until the advent of HIV, medical science even believed that progress was being made. Now with places in the world like Malawi, where 33 percent of pregnant women are already HIV positive, and when some HIV carriers are so infectious and promiscuous that a single index case caused the infection of 13 women and two of their infants,[12] it is clear that this "progress" is too little, too late. All who are in this debate over sex education will admit to the extraordinarily high cost in both dollars and suffering that the STD and HIV epidemics bring. All agree that

11. CDC, "Clusters of HIV-Positive Young Women — New York, 1997-1998," *Morbidity and Mortality Weekly Report* 48 (1999): 413-16.

12. "Clusters of HIV-Positive Young Women — New York, 1997-1998," pp. 413-16.

lifelong monogamy is a 100 percent effective choice, and all agree that anyone can choose it. You don't need to wait for a vaccine or a powerful new antiviral in order to have truly safe sex. True compassion would call for a primary sex education strategy of risk avoidance.

Christians can have a powerful voice in discussing primary strategy for sex education because their perspective is unique. The Christian worldview is unique in that its followers are commanded to demonstrate love and compassion in their actions toward others. In Matthew 5:44 Jesus told his followers, "Love your enemies and pray for those who hate you. Bless those who curse you and do good to those who hate you." The command to show love is in stark contrast to a naturalistic view where survival of the fittest is the operational principle or a feminist view where exercising power and choice can create new groups of disenfranchised individuals. If you were dying from HIV, who would you most like to see — Richard Dawkins, Gloria Steinem, or Mother Teresa? Most people would answer Mother Teresa. Yet Mother Teresa, as a Christian, would lay claim to exclusive truth in very radical terms, terms like these: "I am the way, the truth and the life" (John 14:6). As Christians, our radical truth claims include the sanctity of the sexual union within the bonds of marriage. This truth, as C. S. Lewis once wrote, is so "contrary to our instincts" that the only way it can be understood or accepted is if it is undergirded by love.[13] If it is not undergirded by love it makes the possessor of that truth obnoxious and the dogma expressed becomes repulsive.

Day-to-day examples of that love speak volumes in a postmodern society where self-seeking attitudes run rampant. There are numerous examples. Casa Gloriosa is a home in Tucson, Arizona, for persons infected with HIV and their families. It provides support, encouragement, and love. Casa Gloriosa is well received by the homosexual community, even though Christians run it, because of the compassion given to those who have nothing to give in return. Mother Teresa's work with victims of HIV is another example of that love and compassion.

Christians who participate in the public debate over sexual education need to be known by their love. Love means more than just teaching sexual abstinence. Love means aggressively advocating for STD screening and treatment programs as well. Love means reaching out to those suffering with HIV and touching them in the same way that Jesus touched the lepers of his day. Love means being willing to do the work and to be completely informed with current medical information. Love means being willing to test, evaluate, and do research on sex education programs and submit that work to the peer re-

13. C. S. Lewis, *Mere Christianity* (New York: Simon and Schuster, 1943), p. 90.

view literature so these ideas can enter the public debate. Love also means developing and promoting secondary strategies for specific high-risk groups. This is critical because not all people will choose risk avoidance.

Yet even as we develop and implement secondary prevention and educational strategies such as increased screening and treatment and targeted messages to high-risk groups, the primary strategy should emphasize risk avoidance. The central question becomes: What are we really teaching our youth in this area? "Safe sex" or "saved sex"? But if we choose "safe sex" how safe is safe? Condoms are 90 percent effective for preventing the transmission of HIV. Can you live with a 10 percent chance that your method will fail? And what about HPV? There is currently no clinical medical evidence to suggest that condoms are effective in reducing risk for HPV. Can you live with a prevention method that gives no discernible risk reduction for cervical cancer? Do we want the primary STD prevention message to convey optimal health, or will we settle for less?

Bioethics on the College Campus

Arnold G. Hyndman, Ph.D., and Paul C. Madtes, Jr., Ph.D.

Introduction

Within Western society, colleges and universities are considered the most open and significant arena in the marketplace of ideas. They have a dominant role in influencing society at virtually all levels as they are relied upon for the training of people for citizenship, the workplace, and leadership in nearly every field and endeavor. However, on secular campuses and increasingly on Christian college campuses, the traditional Christian viewpoint is intentionally avoided, restricted, or outright excluded. This should be a matter of grave concern not only to Christians, but to those in academia who truly value the free exchange of ideas and who recognize the importance of such exchanges to democracy, freedom, human understanding, and social well-being.

The exclusion of Christian perspectives from Western colleges and universities has profound social implications because the university is likely the most dominant social institution in the world today. Charles Malik, in his book *A Christian Critique of the University* (Ontario, Canada: North Waterloo Academic Press, 1982), characterized the university as one of the greatest inventions of Western civilization. According to Dr. Malik, the university has more influence on the nature of society than the church, government, economic enterprises, the professions, the media, or even families. His argument for the dominance of the university is based in part on the fact that all these social institutions rely on colleges and universities for the education and training of their leaders, inventors, educators, professionals, administrators and workers, and citizens of every kind. Directly or indirectly, the influence of colleges and universities is pervasive throughout Western civilization today.

Since the Western university is now the model for higher education and training throughout the world, the impact of the university as an institution is global. Thus, the decline of Christian thought within academia has profound implications for a variety of social issues, including bioethics.

To illustrate the influence of the university and its ideas on bioethical issues, it would be instructive to examine the composition of two national bodies that advise the United States government on bioethical issues. The National Bioethics Advisory Committee has seventeen members. Ten of these members are university professors and its chair is a university president. On the National Advisory Council for Human Genome Research, thirteen of the council's seventeen members are university professors. Even though their deliberations are likely to have major implications for a wide segment of society, it is likely that very few in the general public would even consider it inappropriate for those from the university to have an overwhelming domination in consideration of these issues. This is a significant point in a social-political climate that emphasizes representative governance. Professors in the United States represent only two-tenths of one percent of the total population and yet their influence in key areas of bioethics clearly is far beyond their numerical presence. Those who still believe that a Christian viewpoint is critical in the formation of social issues and policies, and in the development of moral and ethical standards, should also understand the importance of having a Christian worldview as a vital part of the intellectual activity that occurs on college and university campuses at all levels.

The challenge is that in society in general, and even with the Christian church, there is a compartmentalization of our spiritual life from other aspects of our lives, both private and public. This is true at secular colleges, but is also true on Christian campuses, which often have the stated mission of preparing people to serve the church and to be "salt and light" to the rest of society. However, a failure to completely integrate one's spiritual life with the other aspects of living has resulted in an inability of Christian colleges to provide deep, consistent, and moral perspectives to many of the issues and insights that have developed within the last several decades. The major objective of Christian colleges ought to be to train students and others to be effective at integrating faith and learning. Christian colleges ought to be at the forefront of societal debate on moral issues like bioethics. Yet, strangely, faculty and students on these campuses are generally unprepared to provide strong intellectual leadership in these key areas.

The purpose of this essay is to present ideas to Christians and others in academia on how they can actively be part of a process to engage the university community with a Christian worldview.

Approaches to Influencing Your Campus

The Secular Campus

George Marsden, in *The Soul of the American University* (New York: Oxford University Press, 1994), observed that the American university system originated in the 1700s from colleges that were Christ-centered in their mission. This Christian influence began to decline during the first few decades of the twentieth century, and became virtually absent by the last few decades of the century. Dr. Joseph Mellichamp, in his book *Ministering in the Secular University* (Carrollton, Tex.: Lewis and Stanley, 1997), suggested that the marginalization of Christianity in the university is a result of Christians not engaging in the fight to keep Christian ideas in the university's marketplace of ideas. The implication of this statement is that those who hold a Christian worldview simply allowed other voices to silence their own. They retreated from academia and thus lost a role in shaping and influencing what has become the dominant institution in the culture. Dr. Mellichamp believes that Christians, having lost a place within academia, must now equip themselves to reclaim what was once commonplace, a voice in the university. To do so, he argues that Christians must understand and expose the hypocrisy of the university that rejects full and fair expression of Christian ideas while embracing virtually every other idea known to humankind. Any complete strategy to make a difference on a college campus should include efforts at the individual, local, regional, and national levels.

One of the unique features of a university community is that nearly every member (faculty, staff, administrators, and students) has a personal desire to be an influence within and outside of the community. Each has, or is developing, a perspective of (1) life and how it should be lived, (2) the world and how it should be organized, (3) thoughts on the nature of social order, and (4) the system of beliefs that should govern it. Therefore, for the Christian interested in bioethics (or any other topic), it is appropriate and consistent with the nature of the university environment for him or her to bring a Christian worldview to bear in influencing both the world within and outside of academia.

It is typical in academic settings for teachers and others to make their worldviews known in the classroom and elsewhere within the community. People will proudly present their identification as a humanist, feminist, socialist, scientist, capitalist, artist, environmentalist, "community activist," evolutionist, and nearly every other "ist" and "ism" that one can imagine. The rare exception is the Christian. Christians have been led to accept the view that, unlike every other system of beliefs that is openly presented in colleges

91

and universities, theirs is a private matter not appropriate for the public realm. They have falsely been informed that the founding principles of modern society prevent religious views from being expressed except in private religious settings. This is not true. There is a healthy tension that exists between the free expression of one's views and the official endorsement of any view by any institution. Within this middle ground there is significant latitude for a vigorous presentation of a Christian worldview within the university environment.

As an individual, the first step is to identify yourself as a Christian, with colleagues, in the classroom, the workplace, and in speaking opportunities. Dr. Mellichamp provides an effective description on how best to do this. Colleges and universities are working and learning environments where values and judgment are important. For the Christian working in a university community, his or her worldview and approach to a discipline and other university work is (or ought to be) influenced by a commitment to Christ. Just as it is common with other background information throughout the university, to identify facts which are likely to influence one's perspectives (such as degrees, schools attended, disciplines studied, the type of work being done, family life), so should a Christian's identification with Christ be made known to those with whom he or she will work and interact. This provides a fair and open context for interacting and engaging others in the marketplace of ideas.

In addition, more public influence can be made by writing letters to the editor of the school paper on various bioethical topics as related to issues on the campus. It might be useful to prepare a series of position papers on a variety of bioethical issues and have them circulated among various colleagues. This could serve as the basis of volunteering to present guest lectures on bioethics in various classes or other public speaking opportunities on the campus and elsewhere.

While a single individual can have a significant impact on a campus, joining forces with one or more like-minded individuals will dramatically increase one's ability to make a difference on a college campus. The most significant role that a colleague will play in this process is encouragement. At times it can be difficult and challenging to present a Christian worldview within the university environment. To have someone who shares your commitment, someone to pray with, to develop strategies with, and to assist in their implementation is critical. Furthermore, efforts of two or more people will grant greater legitimacy to your ideas and will serve to encourage other Christians on campus to likewise be an influence.

Being a member of a university community also allows for the opportunity to make a difference on a regional or national level. In many ways, a consistent and strong regional influence of a Christian perspective in bioethics may be more important than attempting to have a minimal national impact. In addition to letters and articles to professional bioethics journals, letters to local, regional, or national papers and magazines will extend your ability to make a difference beyond the borders of your campus. It is important to understand that being affiliated with a college or university has social and cultural status that will create opportunities and a willingness for people to listen to your ideas. An added benefit of this approach is that as your impact outside your campus community is noticed within academia, your status and influence within your campus community will also increase. This synergy is often overlooked, but is vital in making a difference on your campus. Another important tool is organizing conferences that bring to your campus scholars and others to present their perspective on bioethical issues. This can be a powerful and highly visible means of presenting a Christian perspective that will shape and influence the intellectual and ethical ideas that emanate from your campus.

The Christian Campus

One of the advantages of being in a Christian college environment is the greater opportunity that this setting may provide for directly linking a spiritual perspective to issues present in the discipline. Unfortunately, many faculty in this setting focus on academic development that is limited to content related to specific disciplines and ignore the opportunity to model the integration of faith and learning. As a result, students often complete their academic program without the experience of processing how their Christian worldview impacts their understanding of their discipline and how that affects the application of new knowledge. Since it is imperative that colleges and universities prepare their students for more than entering the professional environment, engaging students in the active exercise of applying knowledge appropriately can facilitate the development of critical thinking skills that will enable these students to become change agents in society. Bioethical issues lend themselves to in-depth consideration in the science, social sciences, and even humanities curriculum.

There are many ways faculty can engage students in the discussion of bioethical issues. Only three will be described here. First, additional readings, questions, and discussions in a variety of science and non-science courses that focus on the consequences for specific scientific discovery on individuals and society can be introduced. The objective is to provide, in multiple courses, training for students to develop critical analysis of implications of thinking and discovery in a wide range of disciplines. One model for doing this is requiring a weekly reading assignment, which is discussed during the last segment of class time at the end of the week (last class session for the week). Students can be required to bring two written questions for discussion, which will be handed in at the end of the discussion. While most questions will not be raised due to time limitations, this approach forces students to complete the assigned reading and begin engaging in thought regarding the issues raised in the reading. Once a student has completed four years as a student, he or she should be able to analyze an issue and critically defend a Christian perspective.

A second approach is to create a seminar series or course on bioethics using current topics found in the newspaper or other popular press. This would be the basis from which to direct a more scholarly examination of a subject with the objective of first developing an understanding of an issue and then learning how to educate others about the issue based on more complete study of the topic. One model for accomplishing this is as follows. The course could be divided into two parts. During the first half, the students would be led through an exercise in learning how to gather information regarding the topic. Then, the information would be analyzed to identify the questions that must be addressed to establish an understanding of the issue. Next, the questions would be ranked in priority to determine which aspects are foundational to the issue and which are not. Finally, the students would build an understanding of the key aspects starting from a Christian worldview. The second half of the course would allow the students to repeat this experience using a new issue. The result is the students learn and practice analyzing issues while integrating their faith and their learning. This provides students with the vitally important skills of effectively preparing others to understand and articulate bioethical issues from a Christian perspective.

A third approach is to establish an annual bioethical conference where a broad cross-section of individuals (for instance, undergraduate students, graduate students, faculty, clinicians, and professionals outside academia) can gather to examine and discuss key bioethical issues. One model of a daylong conference uses keynote addresses, small group discussion of case studies, and question-and-answer sessions to facilitate this process. This approach would enable those involved to be exposed to and trained in a variety of disciplines to develop informed views on bioethical issues, which they could share with others. In addition, the participants would begin to establish contacts with others, enabling ongoing discussion and action on the issues during the coming year. The addition of an evening public presentation could broaden the impact of the conference by engaging individuals who are only marginally interested in bioethical issues and would not participate in a daylong conference.

Challenges to a Christian Influence on College Campuses

Presenting a Christian worldview as a viable perspective in bioethics or other disciplines will generate obstacles and opposition. Some will be personal and others institutional in nature. Although there is almost a limitless list of obstacles and opposition, we present a few as a means to consider the range of possibilities and how best to confront them.

On a personal level some of the obstacles include fear, other priorities, apathy, and limited time. Each of these has some degree of validity and as such can easily derail attempts to bring a Christian worldview into the bioethics debate on campus.

First, fear is probably the greatest factor that prevents the articulation of a Christian worldview on campus, at least by Christians. The concerns are based in part on the real possibility that a bold, clear, and persistent presentation of a Christian worldview could have a negative impact on one's standing within the university community. It is important to remember that truth, even in scholarship, is not achieved without some sacrifice. The greatest antidote to fear is spiritual and intellectual preparation. It is critical that a Christian worldview in bioethics be approached on the university campus with prayer, careful study, and a logical presentation of the argument. Developing and practicing these disciplines within a circle of a small group of supporters is an excellent means for overcoming fear and creating a sound academic presentation that will serve to minimize some of the opposition.

Second, university life can be very demanding. In an age of significant specialization, individuals must devote themselves to the mastery of precise disciplines or tasks. Each person interested in promoting a Christian worldview in bioethics must determine the degree to which this topic will be a part of your activity on campus. This decision should be deliberate. Prioritizing your commitment to promoting this topic will enhance your efficiency. By the same token, your passion for bioethics and particularly a Christian view of the subject may not rate as important to others within the university as it does to you. This should not be discouraging. There are many competing interests on a campus and multiple ideas can flourish at the same time. It is best to develop a presence within a community of interested scholars before attempting to influence a large segment of the university community. This is the way academia conducts itself. Members outside of an area of interest will determine their reaction to an issue based in some measure on the critique of those for whom this is of greater interest. As one is successful in presenting the central and universal issues of a Christian view of bioethics to a small group within the university, then the greater community is more likely to view this as a topic worthy of consideration. Each college and university has a niche of opportunity for the presentation of bioethics. It is within this niche that most of the foundational work must be done. Your first step is to discover that niche. This is true for those who have expertise in bioethics, but lack an affiliation with a college or university. In this case, offering to provide a guest lecture or presentation to a class or seminar can be an exciting opportunity to enrich the curriculum and can serve as an entry to the campus.

Third, often in universities, competing interests create apathy and limit the time that an individual can devote to any topic. One advantage in the area of bioethics is that it is a subject that will likely impact most people directly or indirectly. As a result, the potential for broad, if not sustained, interest in bioethics can be cultivated in most people in the academic community.

Fourth, institutional barriers exist to the presenting of a Christian view of bioethics, including legal limitations, college policies, limited access to institutional resources for scholarly activities, and breaking through the formal barriers that often exist in a classroom setting. One of the most common barriers placed before those who wish to present a Christian perspective on bioethics is the notion that the expression of a Christian viewpoint is a violation of the separation between church and state. Such an interpretation is simply inaccurate. Rather, as clearly presented by John W. Whitehead in *The Freedom of Religious Expression in Public Universities and High Schools* (Westchester, Ill.: Crossway Books, 1985), school administrators and policies cannot regulate the content of ideas that students may speak about or hear, or that teachers may express. Furthermore, because nearly all college and university campuses have become open forums for the expression of a variety of ideas, the rights of free expression are extended to non-students and non-teachers as well. It is important for you to know the facts and be prepared to defend the expression of your convictions, remembering that ideas on campuses can be shared in both formal settings like the classroom and informal gatherings of clubs, organizations, study groups, and lunches. Another challenge in presenting a Christian viewpoint on bioethics is that there may be departmental resistance to using institutional resources for speakers and other scholarly activities that have a Christian focus. This can be overcome by networking with colleagues who have strong academic credentials, finding local Christian bioethicists who may speak on your campus for little or no cost, and most importantly persistently presenting the scholarly content of a Christian perspective in bioethics.

Conclusion

Making a difference on a college or university campus on the topic of bioethics, or any topic, requires a systemic, prayerful, and persistent approach to the presentation of a Christian perspective. The importance of the Western university in the creation, acceptance, and dissemination of ideas makes this a vital objective. Regardless of whether it is a Christian or secular campus, there will be challenges to presenting a strong, clear, and highly visible Christian viewpoint on bioethics. Success will require personal commitment and the support and assistance of others. Our society is in the midst of a biotechnological revolution that will change the very core of Western society and culture. For this reason, an extended presentation of a Christian worldview is essential.

Case Studies

As an aid in thinking about the issues that may confront a person wanting to extend a Christian perspective to bioethics on a college campus, we offer these case studies as an exercise in conceptualizing the various challenges that may arise. Consider how you might handle these various situations on your campus.

Case #1

Progress Versus Respect

A public university has received a private grant of $10 million to establish an embryonic tissue transplant center that promises to make significant progress in treating several human diseases. Recently, two local politicians wrote the president of the university saying that because the new center uses human embryos it does not respect human life and should be closed. The president decides to form a university-wide committee to study the matter and make a recommendation. He has expressed his hope that the committee supports the center and its activities. Because the president is aware of your interest in bioethics you have been asked to serve on this committee. As a member of the committee, what would your position be on this issue? How would you influence the activities of the committee and its outcome?

Case #2

Understanding School Violence, Who Are Experts?

The Department of Sociology is planning to sponsor a symposium on the reasons behind the recent highly publicized violent events on high school campuses. The department chair has indicated that she will invite experts who will be able to provide important insight into this problem including the biology of violence. On her list of speakers are a social biologist, a child psychologist, and the head of the local teachers' union. You write the chair and suggest that a local pastor who runs an after-school program for high school students that includes Bible study and community service would be a valuable speaker at the symposium. The chair answers by saying that your suggestion has been rejected because this symposium is a scholarly event, not a religious or community discussion and that this pastor does not have academic standing that would merit participation in the symposium. How should you respond?

Case #3

Perspective Versus Proselytizing

You are an instructor in the biology department. At the start of each semester you share with your students a little information about yourself which includes the fact that you are a Christian and that your faith is a strong factor in influencing your understanding of biology, particularly issues of bioethics that will be discussed in the course. The readings on bioethics that you assign include some works by Christian scholars and writers. One day your department chair stops by your office to inform you that he has heard that you are proselytizing in your classroom and that you must cease making reference to your religious beliefs and alter your course to remove its religious bias. What should you do?

Case #4

Bioethics in the Classroom

The small Christian college where you are a faculty member encourages integration of faith and learning in the classroom. You decide to introduce discussion of the bioethical implications of scientific discoveries. However, most students come from similar backgrounds and lack experience in addressing issues in depth. They are used to talking about topics that do not require them to consider alternative scenarios. For example, a typical discussion on euthanasia results in the class all stating objections to the taking of life, but no one presents a solid rationale for the position and no one can suggest actions to take. How would you facilitate integration of faith and learning in this environment so that the students develop skill in discussion and learn how to impact the culture in which they live?

Case #5

A Speaker on Bioethics

You serve as a member of a planning committee for bringing guest speakers to campus. Since you are part of a Christian college associated with a specific denomination, you are limited in the range of speakers permitted on campus. While you wish to have a debate on a controversial issue that includes individuals who hold to opposing viewpoints, institutional policy does not permit this. How would you enable the campus community to understand the two sides of the issue?

Case #6

Faculty Involvement

The Christian community has done well at presenting its faith as foundational for living. However, efforts to develop an understanding that rhetoric is insufficient have not been as successful. Therefore, you wish to prepare undergraduate students at your Christian college to impact both the church and the secular communities into which they are going upon graduation. You seek to involve other faculty members across campus, crossing disciplines. However, there is a general apathy toward the idea, indicating others do not feel that their involvement is essential. How would you move forward?

The Media and Its Opportunities

Teri N. Goudie

Dispelling Two Myths

The media is not out to get you. Any investigative reporter would tell you that you would fail to find anyone in the backroom of a news station or newspaper plotting to control the news. They do not plot against you. So, let's dispel that myth right now. Today, news organizations are driven by numbers. At this moment there is a group of people at Disney, in New York, looking at white pieces of paper deciding where they can cut costs in order to make a profit. They are not out to get you. They are out to get viewers.

The other myth to dispel is this: you cannot change the system. However, you may not be able to change the system but you can make a personal difference. I learned this lesson in the pro-life movement. I got frustrated constantly asking, "When are we going to overturn this decision?" and "When is this gonna happen?" Eventually my colleagues and I realized that it may not happen in our lifetimes, but maybe in our children's lifetimes. We can make a difference. We can help those in need.

The Necessity of a Method

This chapter presents a method that will help you make a difference through the media. Physicians know the value of a good surgical method. Pastors know the value of a well-prepared sermon. This chapter will give you a methodology to use each and every day with the issues that matter to you most. It will allow you to have a place at the table, to make news and not just noise, and to turn words into action. Begin in your hospital and with your local newspaper.

This method can also be applied to everything else you are doing: presentations, meetings, and one-on-one conversations. You can use this method in everything you do: on grand rounds, speaking to your family, or giving a speech. Consider this method as a good golf swing. Embrace it on every course, with every player, in every type of wind condition and you will win.

The Method

This method centers on the way a presentation for the media is prepared. It's all in the preparation, the back-swing. This chapter will demonstrate to you a five-step method of preparation that will allow you to influence the editing, ensure that you get your point across, control a reporter's pre-sought agenda, and guarantee that you make news — not noise. The back-swing consists of five simple steps that take only two minutes to implement. You do not need to spend two hours preparing for a media interview. Two minutes, done correctly, is sufficient. The quality of the preparation is much more critical than the quantity.

Step one: Focus on the audience, not the reporter. A common mistake is allowing the reporter to control the agenda, only answering the questions the reporter poses. People often wait for reporters to take them to the right place. Too much time is spent trying to ascertain an interviewer's motivation, nearly forgetting about the person they are really trying to reach. In a recent interview, I might have surprised the interviewer a bit because I sat in the chair sounding like the media coach I am before I even let her turn on the microphone. Immediately, I asked, "Who is listening to the program right now?" "What do you think they are interested in knowing?" and "Who did you talk to right before I came to the microphone?" The answers to these questions gave me a lot of leverage in that interview. I wasn't just talking to the interviewer. I targeted my comments towards the audience. If I had simply answered the questions and gone no further, the interviewer, not me, the media expert, would have controlled the agenda.

So, remember: When you appear on "60 Minutes" you are not speaking only to Mike Wallace. If you only go as far as Mike Wallace, you will get nothing out of that opportunity. You are speaking to the fifty-eight-year-old couple who sit home on Sunday night to watch "60 Minutes." What do they really care about? That is the audience focus I want you to have. And with that focus you have just unleashed your power with the media.

You actually have more power than a reporter. On a daily, hourly, weekly basis you are far closer to the patients, residents, and customers than, as a reporter, I will ever be. These are the people I am trying to sell my newspaper to — your patients, the people in the communities. I am not out there every Saturday morning talking to people about the issue, trying to persuade people, but you are. If you begin my interview with that piece that only you hear on a daily basis, I will write your story. I know, as a reporter, that is what people are going to talk about tomorrow morning in the back of the bus. I may even use the story to lead the news that night. It will make a tremendous difference for you.

It's a pronoun switch. Do not speak to the media through your eyes as the advocate — that seems obvious. Do not even speak about your eyes as an organization or a hospital. Speak about the issues consistently through the eyes of the people who are really driving the decision. If you consistently talk about the issue through the "you" perspective, as opposed to the "me" or the "we" perspective, you will be able to much better control what is written or reported. That is the power you bring to the media encounter.

Step two: Always speak top-down. The most important information first. It is crucial for you to always speak in a way that connects to the way people listen today. People today generally have a hard time processing information because there is so much to be processed. We are no longer passive recipients. We actively pursue what we want to know, listening for the headline first. This is a tremendous challenge to those of you who are trained as physicians, lawyers, and scientists. Law and medical school trained you to do it just the opposite. When you write a piece for *JAMA* you outline the hypothesis, the methodology, and then the conclusion. When you are presenting a case, you build your case and then supply the bottom line.

That is opposite of the way you should be speaking to the media. That is why doctors often get misquoted and many scientists never get a chance to speak to an issue. They often answer a reporter's questions by putting their conclusions at the end. There is a physical problem here: when they are at their conclusion the reporter is still back on the third point they made. When the reporter goes to write the piece, he or she finds notes full of sentence fragments. You risk being unintentionally misquoted, simply because, as the reporter, I cannot legibly write down a lot of information that I do not understand. I want you to start with your conclusion. Not only does that allow you to provide a more direct quote, it no longer matters if you are cut off, as you have already stated your conclusion. It also makes you the context provider — this is very, very important today.

Would anybody read the play-by-play of the Cubs game without looking at the score first? No. Would anybody watch the U.S. Open without the leader board in the upper-left-hand corner? No. Without it you have no context. You are not going to let the doctor treat you without him telling you whether it will hurt or not. We all listen for the headline first. Without it, we stop listening. Therefore, if you are speaking top-down through the media, you are now going to drive the context. As a reporter, I will come back to you for further comment because I know you are the person who can frame it for me and help me understand it better.

Step three: Always speak in terms of answering the unmet question. Anticipate the question before an interview. I am not referring to the questions you are going to get from the reporters. That is a waste of time, since they often ask you the same questions. Focus on the unanswered questions of the people in the audience. What are those questions? What are those unmet needs and what are you doing to solve them? Nobody is going to invest their time, their money, or their support based on what happened yesterday or what you are doing today. Rather, we invest our time, our money, and support based on what you are doing to solve tomorrow's unmet needs. That is what the media is looking for. That is what drives the stock market. You do not buy stock in a company based on what the company did yesterday — you want to know what is going to happen tomorrow. Thus, when you are asked to comment on the issues, I highly suggest you think about, not just addressing the pain of yesterday, but giving very specific ways that we can build for tomorrow. That is what will bring them to your side of the table — just like it did for Michael Jordan. When Michael Jordan got hurt, when he got caught gambling, when he retired, he did not lose one corporate sponsor. He always did it through the eyes of the people who were really driving the decisions: the guy on the South Side of Chicago who paid seventy-five bucks to take his kid to a game. You want to talk to the media about the issue in terms of a solution to an unmet need. Not many people realize that there are alternatives to fetal tissue research. I am sure that there are many people that would yearn for that kind of alternative, but if nobody presents it as a solid alternative to an unmet need, few people will recognize the solution.

Answer this unmet question by using comparisons. The number one way to predict what the quote is going to be or the sound bite is to recognize that they will always quote the comparison. I challenge you to pick up the newspaper and a red pen and circle every quote; listen to the news and note every sound bite. It is almost always a comparison. There is no coincidence here. If you switch from channel two to five to seven — they all use the same sound bite from Mayor Daley. They all pick the same thing that President Clinton said. There is no science here. The media always picks the comparison. People like President Clinton learned long ago how to drive the quote and control the media — by speaking in sound bites, by speaking in comparisons.

What do I mean by comparisons? Imagine that your local news station is doing a piece on a pro-choice rally, and you are asked to comment. How can you control which comment they pick? If you say something like, "You know, for every six pro-choice people out here today, there are 60 pro-life women in the western suburbs of Chicago, who, as we speak, are gathering diapers to help women with problem pregnancies." They will have to quote that. Not only is it compelling, but it is a comparison. Everyone who hears that will talk about it tomorrow morning.

Think about the quotes you remember from history: "Ask not what your country can do for you . . ." "One small step . . ." Research indicates that the new pieces of information that people remember on a daily basis are the pieces that somebody has attached to what you already know. That's how you teach. You can teach through the media using comparison. Attach your ideas to something already known, drawn through comparisons. Formulate these comparisons before you speak to a reporter.

Step four: Before you speak, you need one core theme. No longer can you go into a presentation, a meeting, or an interview with three message points. As good as a speaker is, people only remember 10 percent of what is said. Whatever people talk about during the coffee break is what will be remembered. We need to ensure that when we speak, everything we say is attached to one core thing. No matter what you talked about in the coffee break, a core theme was part of it. You can have three messages, but they need to be attached to a greater theme. If you have one core theme for a presentation or an interview, suddenly the editing process doesn't matter anymore. It doesn't matter what I, as the reporter, put in the lead. If your core theme is a part of everything you say, you get to control what reporters write. You can control the headlines.

If you have one consistent theme to come back to when you have been asked difficult questions, whether you're on radio, television, speaking to a local reporter, or on a panel discussion, you become a personal, living example of consistency, believability, and trust. People will walk away, perhaps not remembering what you said, but remembering that you were consistent. People trust consistency. That is how President Clinton got elected: He kept going back to that same theme. He would go into the town-hall meetings, saying things like, "I know the price of bread, and I know that Susie over there is worried about her kids going to school tomorrow morning. And I know you need three thousand new police officers. It all comes down to the economy."

Even though he rarely kept those promises, at the time people believed he was actually going to do something.

Let me give you another example of the importance of maintaining a core theme. Ten years ago, I trained a gentleman for United Airlines in Chicago. I trained him before the Sioux City, Iowa, crash. That was that plane that cartwheeled on the tarmac. It happened at 3:30 P.M. on a Friday. At 5:00 P.M. United was holding a press conference despite the fact that their legal counsel warned, "You can't do this. Rumors, speculation, liability!" United answered, "Maybe, but if we don't get out there and show the world that we're going to be the source of information on this issue, someone else is going to speak for us." They obviously did not want that to happen. This gentleman handled a very aggressive group of reporters for forty-five minutes in that press conference, and then they kept broadcasting him for almost twenty-four hours. Nonetheless, if you were sitting at home with your families you would hear one core theme, "We care. Family."

What can we learn from this? Two things. First, United recognized that the audience was not the reporters. Many reporters knew more than United did. In order to control that media environment, United had to go beyond the reporters. They had to go to you and me sitting at home, where we were wondering if we knew anybody on the plane and wondering if we were safe to fly tomorrow morning. They went directly to your unmet need and wanted to show control and stability. They did it by empowering the gentleman to have one core theme to come back to, no matter what. He became a living example of the control and stability. He did not have to say it; you walked away with that image.

The other thing United recognized was that it would have been very easy for the world to react to "UAL, the big conglomerate." People are more likely to forgive a person than a conglomerate. By putting a face on the issue, United gave us a way to forgive them. It is all about people. We heard about the heroic pilot the next day. I can easily criticize a conglomerate, a movement, or an association, but it is really hard to criticize the people being affected by the issues. If you put yourself on the right side of the issues and put a face on the issues, you may not be victorious tomorrow, you may not be victorious next week, but you are leaving behind a mark, a definite mark, and the way you do that is not only to have that one core theme but to go to the next and final step.

Step five: You have to prove it! You have to have good, vivid support and examples.

- Paint the pictures that you want people to see. Few people remember the words that you speak. Rather, they remember the pictures you compel them to see. Thus, the media is a marvelous opportunity to paint the pictures that are going to compel the right actions. Paint pictures for tomorrow, not yesterday. The pictures for tomorrow will compel me to make my decision. Localize your pictures. If you give a newspaper reporter a local example from your community, it will get used, because again, you are giving him or her the piece that people are talking about in the back of the bus.

- Tell stories. If you look back on recent events in the news, you will recognize that it became far easier for people in our country to understand a simple lie than it was a complex truth. Through the media, take your complex truth and present it in a simple form. One of the best ways to do that is through a story. We learned long ago that when Mary Tyler Moore talks about diabetes, and Christopher Reeve talks about spinal disability, people become aware, stereotypes fall, and funding increases. Consider the power of one simple story. A doctor-psychologist being interviewed on the use of Prozac on children was continually interrupted as he let the interviewers control the interview. However, when given a chance, he finally redeemed himself with the power of a story about a specific child's experiences with and without Prozac. The audience he should have remembered he was talking to in the first place consisted of parents who might ask, "What if this was my kid?" The power of the story finally worked for him.

- Use analogy, another positive approach. I train a lot of the medical deans through the Association of American Medical Colleges. I was in Washington doing a session, and the executive director of the association needed some quick help. Ted Koppel had invited him to be on "Nightline" and talk about residency programs. He had been asked, "Is it true that patients are dying because residents are being forced to work 36-hour shifts?!" He wanted to talk about monitoring and accreditation. I suggested that he find a way to put this in perspective for mom and pop in their pajamas, because they would be the audience.

When questioned about the efficiency of students who work these long hours, he used a simple and effective analogy. He explained that students often need to be involved in the entire process of the disease in order to understand it. He compared it to seeing a movie. People cannot go into a movie and understand the entire plot. They need to see the beginning, middle, and end in order to understand it completely. He went on to say, "We want our physicians to ultimately understand when they run into a case that they have seen before that they have to see the whole story, so they can understand it from the piece that they have before them. But it takes experience, and it takes ability to see the whole case unfold in order to gain that kind of experience that you and I want from our doctors. . . ." That is the power of analogy.

- Use numbers, cases, and studies. Of course, you want to have this all ready to go, but be smart about the numbers you use. Try to localize numbers whenever possible. All news is local news. Personalize those numbers. You and I will be exposed to hundreds of numbers today. The only numbers we will actually remember when we go to sleep tonight are the numbers that had a face on them. If you miss your 7:05 flight back home, you will remember that number. If it takes you an hour and two minutes to drive from here to Chicago, you will remember that number. My kid hits a triple tonight in the sixth inning: I will remember that number. What you can do to drive the numbers that you know are the most important is to put a face to those numbers. For example, it is not 72 percent; it is seven out of ten women who live in Deerfield, Illinois. Put a face on your numbers when you speak to the media. Not only are they more likely to quote those numbers, but people will remember those numbers. Those numbers are more easily catalogued in their mind, plus it allows you to personalize the issue.
- Use third-party endorsement. That means outside sources endorsing your point of view. Credentialed sources are very important today. Listen for the specifics, document them, and have a media file in your desk. People want specifics, and it is the specifics that work.

Let me describe to you one last example implementing all five steps. A case in Illinois involved my client, Motorola. A woman driving her sick child to the doctor reached down to answer her phone. She lost control of her car and killed a man. The man's family pressed charges and the mother ended up in jail. They also filed a lawsuit and found a legislator who wrote a bill that would require people to pull over before using cell phones. My client, Motorola, was naturally affected by the issue. After the media presented a tape of weeping and unanswered questions, they sought out the blame, going to the industry to see what they had to say about the problem. The industry was ready. The gentleman who spoke on behalf of Motorola, a third-party person, decided that instead of being defensive and reactive, he was going to use this as a chance to teach. So he used this five-step method, and became the listener's advocate in the interview. He responded to the interviewer's questions regarding the use of cell phones by focusing on the fact that they are highly recognized as an important safety tool. He began with a word of sympathy, a good way to disarm an enemy in a media interview. He spoke top-down to his audience, answering unmet questions of safety by explaining that 98,000 times each day someone uses the cell phone to call for help, report accidents, save lives, and stop crimes. The gentleman agreed that answering a cell phone while driving is a case of judgment just as many other things people do behind the wheel. This gentleman had an effective interview.

*   *   *

When you speak to the media, you speak top-down, not bottom-up, with the audience focus in mind, giving a solution to an unmet need, and wonderful proof material, all consistent with your central theme. It only takes you two minutes to pull it together. A common thread throughout this preparation method, this golf swing, is that you are always golfing with the end-consumer in mind, whether that's the woman, the man, the patient — you are always speaking as a community advocate.

In addition to the five-step method, here a few suggestions:

- Control your delivery. When speaking to a print reporter on the phone, stand up. I am affected by the enthusiasm of your voice when you are on the phone with me. Stand up!
- Remember that there is no such thing as "off the record." Everything you say is subject to be used. Most reporters will not let you see the article before it is printed, but they will call you to check a quote. Give them your number if you want them to call you and check back with you.
- Do not do an interview longer than twenty minutes. After twenty minutes you will get tired.
- When you speak on the radio, remember that your voice is important. Sit on the edge of your seat. Use your hands, and paint pictures because radio listeners want to be able to see it. It is a great chance to visualize. When you go to a radio program, always give people a place that they can go to for more information, especially when you are doing the call-in programs. You do not want to get stuck in a two-hour debate with one particular caller. You want to be able to send that caller someplace else for information.
- When on television, appearance really counts. Smiling pleasantly applies to your print and radio interviews as well. If you are smiling on the phone, I can hear it in your voice.
- Only look people in the eye. Do not look at the camera, or you will look like Ross Perot. I felt as if he was using the camera to get to me. The ex-

ception to the rule, the only time you look at a lens, is if you do "Night-line," or a similar remote interview situation with only you and a camera. If there is a person there, you speak to a person. Do not attempt to look away, because your eyes tell me the story.

- Use your hands. If you grip the podium, your voice is going to get very boring because you are not allowing your vocal chords to do their job. Loosen up and visualize by using your hands. Not only is your face more interesting, but your vocal chords are allowed to do their job. You will get inflection. Pausing will make you interesting. Always use your hands. If you are thinking about what you are doing with your hands, you are not thinking about your content.

- Avoid "upspeak," or raising your voice at the end of a sentence. When teenagers use it at the end of each statement, you know something funny is going on. What they are saying is, "Do you believe me? Is this working, mom?" I want you to be definitive and come down at the end of your statements when you speak to the media or give a presentation. Really punctuate at the end for consistency and believability.

- Choice of words is important. Avoid excessive jargon. Do not use acronyms that people do not understand. You will not be quoted if you are using language that I cannot easily share with my audience.

- Do not take ownership for what you do not own. Avoid speaking for the opposition and getting sucked into what I call the David versus Goliath story, us versus them. If the interview centers around "you versus them," you lose the chance to educate people on the realities of the issue.

- Stay on course with a control technique called bridging — going from what they are asking you to what you really think is the most important for the audience to hear. However, you must answer the question first. A lot of politicians think you can just ignore the question and replace it with something else. You can answer the question with "Yes," "No," "I do not know," or "I don't know, but what I do know is this. . . ." You can then go back to what is really most important for your audience.

- Prompt questions. Before you are on a local radio show, write down three good questions you have heard from people in that community. Tell the reporters, "You know, I thought you might be interested in seeing three of the toughest questions we have heard in the last month from the people who are listening to your show." The reporters will love you for that. An example of a phrase you could use: "Again, the one thing I hear every single day from the women in this community is . . ." Continue returning to your main point with phrases like that.

- Make news not just noise, and you will turn words into action. First and foremost, if you speak as the advocate for your community, everything else should eventually fall into place.

In conclusion, this method is practical, it works, and it is designed to make your job of speaking to the media easier. Putting it into practice will enable you to communicate with the media more effectively.

PART III

LAW AND PUBLIC POLICY

Is Statecraft Soulcraft?
Faith, Politics, and Legal Neutrality

Francis J. Beckwith, Ph.D.

[A]bsolute tolerance is altogether impossible; the allegedly absolute tolerance turns into ferocious hatred of those who stated clearly and most forcefully that there are unchangeable standards founded on the nature of man and the nature of things.

Leo Strauss, *Liberalism Ancient and Modern*

It is fashionable today in evangelical circles to speak of the theological posture of Western civilization, and American intellectual culture in particular, as post-Christian. Our most important, influential, and culture-shaping institutions and professions — law, medicine, education, science, media, and the arts — no longer accept the presuppositions of the biblical worldview as part of their philosophical frameworks. Thus, for example, it is not unusual — in fact, it is quite common — to hear academic luminaries from different disciplines in assorted venues defend the right to abortion, same-sex marriage, physician-assisted suicide, as well as policies in education and science (especially in biomedical research) that presuppose naturalism and the political and social theories that flow from it.[1] The ease by which these positions

---

1. *Naturalism* is a philosophical, not scientific, perspective that maintains that the material world is all that exists. All non-natural things like God, angels, souls, or morality do not exist. (Morality, some naturalists argue, is *real*, only insofar as it is a social construc-

are presented, and the absence of a call to justify them by the same standards of philosophical rigor that are required of their opposition, is testimony to how potently naturalism has shaped the ideas, opinions, and policies of those who occupy the seats of cultural influence in our society.

Although few in the evangelical community would dispute the accuracy of this assessment, it is not always clear how a Christian citizen, especially an academic, ought to engage this cultural reality. There is a tendency among evangelical leaders, especially those who wield influence in conservative circles on political and social concerns, to look at challenges to the biblical worldview in a piecemeal fashion, that is, on an issue by issue basis. Although I largely agree with the positions taken by these leaders, in this essay I will suggest another way to look at cultural engagement, one that is the result of employing the resources of philosophical reflection.

Evangelicals seem aware intuitively that in the conflict over cultural values there is not a level playing field. Perspectives that appear antithetical to the biblical worldview seem to be treated by cultural elites as default positions for which no argument or case is required. Proponents for these positions present them as if they were "neutral," "non-sectarian," and "tolerant," while asserting or implying that those who disagree are promoting what is "bigoted," "sectarian," and "intolerant," and consequently, unworthy of serious consideration in our civic culture. But the differences between the biblical worldview and its secular rival cannot be delineated so easily. The latter, I will argue, is just as non-neutral as the former, and for that reason ought not to have the presumption in the public square. In order to illustrate this, we will first look at what I mean by the "biblical worldview" and then move on to political liberalism, the dominant view among secular intellectuals in the West, which is proposed as a neutral political and legal framework in our pluralistic society. After that we will see how political liberalism's alleged neutrality cannot withstand critical scrutiny when applied to particular public policy issues in education, science, and civil liberties.

---

tion resulting from evolution, but it has no ontological status apart from the institutions, laws, and social contracts that have benefited human survival.) Darwinian and Neo-Darwinian evolutionary theory presupposes the truth of naturalism since it denies that an Intelligent Designer had any part as an agent in the creation, sustenance, or history of the world.

I. The Biblical Worldview

What I mean by the "biblical worldview" is the philosophical tapestry of interdependent ideas, principles, and metaphysical claims that are derived from the Hebrew-Christian Scriptures as well as the creeds, theologies, communities, ethical norms, and institutions that have flourished under the authority of these writings. These beliefs are not mere utterances of private religious devotion, but are propositions whose proponents claim accurately instruct us on the nature of the universe, human persons, human communities, and the moral life. The following is a summary of some of these beliefs.[2]

First, there exists an eternally self-existing moral agent named God, who created the universe *ex nihilo*. The universe is completely and absolutely contingent upon God for its beginning, as well as its continued existence. He is, among other things, personal, omnipotent, omniscient, omnipresent, perfectly good, necessary, and infinitely wise.[3] God is not only the Creator of the visible and physical universe, but he is also the source of the invisible and non-physical one. He is the creator of human souls and the ontological source of the moral law, logic, and mathematics.

Second, God created human beings in his image. A human being is not merely a collection of physical parts, but has an underlying unity or soul.[4] A human being's life is sacred from the moment that human being comes into existence; the value of a human being is not something acquired when he or she reaches a certain level of physical complexity, as many secular thinkers maintain.[5] Because human beings are moral agents, they have the capacity to make decisions and judgments within the larger framework of family and community. Thus, for the biblical worldview, marriage, government, and church are not merely social constructs that can be shaped in any way consistent with some utopian political theory. Rather, they are natural insti-

---

2. This is merely a brief summary of my take on the biblical worldview; it is not meant to be an exhaustive presentation and defense of my perspective. I understand that there are intramural disputes among Christians on a number of these points.

3. For a biblical defense of these attributes, see Francis J. Beckwith, "Appendix D: Why the Classical Concept of God Is Biblical," in *See the Gods Fall: Four Rivals to Christianity* by Francis J. Beckwith and Stephen E. Parrish (Joplin, Mo.: College Press, 1997).

4. For a philosophical defense of this viewpoint from a biblical perspective, see J. P. Moreland and Scott B. Rae, *Body and Soul* (Downers Grove, Ill.: InterVarsity Press, 2000).

5. For a critique of this viewpoint, and a defense of what I believe is the biblical one, see Francis J. Beckwith, *Politically Correct Death: Answering the Arguments for Abortion Rights* (Grand Rapids: Baker, 1993). See also, Patrick Lee, *Abortion and Unborn Human Life* (Washington, D.C.: The Catholic University of America Press, 1996); and Moreland and Rae, *Body and Soul.*

tutions in which and by which human beings ought to learn what is good, true, and beautiful. They are part of the furniture of the universe and their continued existence is essential to maintaining the moral ecology of human society. Thus, the end of the community should be to produce good citizens, and therefore, provide a privileged position for these natural institutions.[6]

Third, God reveals himself both in special revelation (2 Tim. 3:14-17), the Bible, as well as general revelation. Concerning the former, if the Bible is truly God's Word, then it must be inerrant, for God himself is perfect (Mark 10:18; Heb. 6:18), and it follows logically that his Word must be as well. The Bible provides us with (1) an account of humanity's genesis and fall, (2) a history of God's chosen people, (3) the institution of the law of Moses and its inadequacy to redeem, (4) prophecy, prayer, wisdom, and poetry, and (5) the good news and story of the first coming of the Messiah and the establishing of his church on earth.

According to Scripture, God has not left himself without a witness among pagans (Acts 14:17). This is called general revelation, since it is something that all people have the capacity to access through observation, reason, and reflection apart from the Bible. J. Budziszewski outlines the five forms in which general revelation is presented in Scripture:

> (1) [T]he testimony of creation, which speaks to us of a glorious, powerful and merciful Creator (Ps. 19:1-6; Acts 14:17; Rom. 1:20); (2) the fact that we are made in the image of God, which not only gives us rational and moral capacities but tells us of an unknown Holy One who is different from our idols (Gen. 1:26-27; Acts 17:22-23); (3) the facts of our physical and emotional design, in which a variety of God's purposes are plainly manifest (Rom. 1:26-27); (4) the law of conscience, written on the heart, which, like the law of Moses, tells us what sin is but does not give us power to escape it (Rom. 2:14-15); (5) the order of causality, which teaches us by linking every sin with consequences (Prov. 1:31).[7]

The fact that Scripture teaches the reality of what has come to be known as general revelation (or natural law, when pertaining to morality) does not mean that one must be a Christian in order to either recognize or have knowledge of it. For example, commonsense appeals to justice, fairness, re-

6. See Kenneth L. Grasso, "Man, Society, and the State: A Catholic Perspective," in *Caesar's Coin Revisited: Christians and the Limits of Government*, ed. Michael Cromartie (Grand Rapids: Eerdmans; Washington, D.C.: Ethics & Public Policy Center, 1996).

7. J. Budziszewski, *Written on the Heart: The Case for Natural Law* (Downers Grove, Ill.: InterVarsity, 1997), pp. 180-81.

spect, and integrity, though employed by citizens who may not share the biblical worldview (or even a broadly theistic worldview), are perfectly legitimate, even though the objective truth of such moral notions seems more compatible with a theistic worldview than a naturalist (or atheistic) one. For example, Plato's critique of moral relativism (see *The Gorgias* and *The Republic*), though not appealing to Scripture, supports a view of morality consistent with the biblical worldview.

We now turn to political liberalism and how it can be employed to restrict the biblical worldview from influencing and shaping our society and its institutions.

II. Political Liberalism

The dominant school of thought in political philosophy today is political liberalism, which is embraced in different forms by a diversity of thinkers.[8] Proponents of political liberalism maintain that the individual has the right,

---

8. Among the diverse proponents of political liberalism (and their representative writings) are John Rawls (*Political Liberalism* [New York: Columbia University Press, 1993]); Ronald Dworkin ("Liberalism," in his *A Matter of Principle* [Cambridge, Mass.: Harvard University Press, 1985]); Thomas Nagel ("Personal Rights and Public Space," *Philosophy and Public Affairs* 24 [1995]); Robert Nozick (*Anarchy, State, and Utopia* [New York: Basic Books, 1974]); Robert Audi ("The Separation of Church and State and the Obligation of Citizenship," *Philosophy and Public Affairs* 18 [1989], and "The Place of Religious Argument in a Free and Democratic Society," *San Diego Law Review* 30 [1993]); and Bruce Ackerman (*Social Justice and the Liberal State* [New Haven, Conn.: Yale University Press, 1980]). There have been a number of critiques of political liberalism. Among them are the following: Michael Sandel, *Liberalism and the Limits of Justice* (New York: Cambridge, 1982); Michael Sandel, *Democracy's Discontent* (Cambridge, Mass.: Harvard University Press, 1996); George Sher, *Beyond Neutrality* (New York: Cambridge, 1997); John Finnis, "Public Reason, Abortion, and Cloning," *Valparaiso University Law Review* 32.2 (Spring 1998); Robert P. George, *Making Men Moral: Civil Liberties and Public Morality* (New York: Oxford, 1993); Robert P. George, "Public Reason and Political Conflict: Abortion and Homosexuality," *Yale Law Journal* 106 (June 1997); Nicholas Wolterstorff, "Why We Should Reject What Liberalism Tells Us about Speaking and Acting in Public for Religious Reasons," in *Religion and Contemporary Liberalism*, ed. Paul J. Weithman (Notre Dame: University of Notre Dame Press, 1997); and J. L. A. Garcia, "Liberal Theory, Human Freedom, and the Politics of Sexual Morality," in *Religion and Contemporary Liberalism*.

For an outstanding debate between two Christian philosophers on this matter, see Audi and Wolterstorff, *Religion in the Public Square* (Lanham, Md.: Rowman & Littlefield, 1997). For a Christian analysis of the notion of equality found in liberal theory, see Louis P. Pojman, "A Critique of Contemporary Egalitarianism: A Christian Perspective," *Faith and Philosophy* 8, no. 4 (October 1991).

within the framework of a liberal democracy, to make choices, unencumbered by another's vision of the good life, based on her preferences which may include moral, philosophical, and religious beliefs. Thus, the state should remain neutral on matters religious and philosophical.

There is another aspect of this version of political liberalism: the secular reason requirement. Its proponents affirm that citizens should not support their public policy proposals by appealing to exclusively religious reasons if they are trying to limit the liberty of other citizens. Consequently, in order to participate in public discourse, the religious person must be willing to supplement his case by citing reasons that are not based on any theological commitment whatsoever. Just as the state must remain neutral on matters of religion, the religious person must provide non-sectarian, or neutral, reasons for matters of state.

The most influential philosopher of political liberalism is John Rawls. His thought, and those of his disciples and allies (including Ronald Dworkin), has had a profound impact on the culture-shaping disciplines of law and political science, especially in the areas of jurisprudence and constitutional theory. According to Rawls, a state (or government) is just if it is the result of principles people would have arrived at if they knew nothing about what they are or what they will become (in other words, whether they are rich or poor, black or white, homosexual or heterosexual, short or tall, male or female).[9] To employ Rawls's terminology, the principles of justice are those agreed to by parties in "the original position" (an imaginary time and place where there is no government) behind "a veil of ignorance" (an imaginary situation in which nobody has any personal knowledge of themselves or their futures). In other words, the principles of justice are those arrived at by means of a social contract that all the "unbiased" parties would agree on so that they can receive full political and social freedom and a minimum standard of financial entitlement just in case it turns out one is, for example, not well off, not naturally gifted, or holds unpopular political or religious opinions. This means that Rawls's principles of justice have little or nothing to do

---

9. Rawls, *Political Liberalism*, pp. 22-28. Rawls's two principles of justice are:

a. Each person has an equal claim to a fully adequate scheme of basic rights and liberties, which scheme is compatible with the same scheme for all; and in this scheme the equal political liberties, and only those liberties, are to be guaranteed their fair value.

b. Social and economic inequalities are to satisfy two conditions: first, they are to be attached to positions and offices open to all under conditions of fair equality of opportunity; and second, they are to be to the greatest benefit of the least advantaged members of society (Rawls, *Political Liberalism*, pp. 5-6).

with the good, the true, or the beautiful. They are principles for ensuring economic entitlement as well as for preventing conflict between individuals each pursuing his or her own subjective view of the good. They are rules for protecting one's interests as well as refereeing the conflicts which result from individuals exercising their autonomy.[10]

According to Rawls, "no comprehensive doctrine is appropriate as a political conception."[11] A doctrine is comprehensive for Rawls "when it includes conceptions of what is of value in human life, and ideals of personal character, as well as ideals of friendship and familial and associational relationships, and much else that is to inform our conduct, and in the limit to our life as a whole."[12] To his credit, Rawls maintains that both religious and philosophical perspectives can be comprehensive doctrines. Although he claims that his view of state neutrality does not prevent proponents of comprehensive doctrines from influencing public policy, their proposals must not be in conflict with the principles of justice (which are the basis, according to Rawls, of constitutional rights) and they must provide publicly accessible reasons (in other words, secular reasons) for their positions.[13] According to Rawls, "Political liberalism sees its form of political philosophy as having its own subject mat-

---

10. Rawls probably would not agree entirely with my depiction of his view, for he considers his theory of justice to be deontological and not utilitarian or egoistic. He writes in one place that his principles of justice, like Immanuel Kant's, are categorical imperatives (Rawls, *Theory of Justice*, p. 253). However, some scholars, such as Sandel (*Liberalism and the Limits of Justice*), J. P. Moreland (in "Rawls and the Kantian Interpretation," in *Simon Greenleaf Review of Law and Religion* 8 [1988-89]), and Keith Pavlischek (*John Courtney Murray and the Dilemma of Religious Toleration* [Kirksville, Mo.: Thomas Jefferson University Press, 1994], pp. 208-12), have made assessments of Rawls's theory which are similar to mine.

11. Rawls, *Political Liberalism*, p. 115.

12. Rawls, *Political Liberalism*, p. 13.

13. See Rawls, *Political Liberalism*, pp. 195-211. There are those to Rawls's political right, such as secular libertarians, who espouse state "neutrality" when it comes to questions of "the good." For example, libertarian social philosopher Murray Rothbard writes: "[W]hile the behavior of plants and at least the lower animals is determined by their biological nature or perhaps by their 'instincts,' the nature of man is such that *each individual person must, in order to act, choose his own ends and employ his own means in order to attain them.* Possessing no automatic instincts, each man must learn about himself and the world, *use his mind to select values,* learn about cause and effect, and act purposively to maintain himself and advance his life. . . . Since each individual must think, learn, value, and choose his or her ends and means in order to survive and flourish, the right of self-ownership gives man the right to perform these vital activities without being hampered and restricted by coercive molestation" (emphasis added) (Murray N. Rothbard, *For a New Liberty: The Libertarian Manifesto*, rev. ed. [San Francisco: Fox & Wilkes, 1978], pp. 28-29).

ter: how is a just and free society possible under conditions of deep doctrinal conflict with no prospect of resolution?" His answer is state neutrality: "To maintain impartiality between comprehensive doctrines, [political liberalism] does not specifically address the moral topics on which those doctrines divide."[14]

Although Rawls believes the philosophical case for his principles of justice succeeds, he understands that for political liberalism to be the ground of a stable and enduring society of competing comprehensive doctrines, each proponent must conclude that Rawls's principles of justice are reasonable from his perspective. This is what Rawls calls an "overlapping consensus." "Thus," according to Rawls, "political liberalism looks for a political conception of justice that we hope can gain the support of an overlapping consensus of reasonable religious, philosophical, and moral doctrines in a society regulated by it."[15] Given this, it is difficult to see how non-liberal positions on issues such as same-sex marriage, physician-assisted suicide, and abortion can even get a hearing in such a state, because those who oppose these practices out of principle usually do so on the basis of some view of human nature and the good life that is not found in Rawls's principles of justice.[16]

III. A Critique of Political Liberalism

It is apparent to any observer of contemporary political discourse that most public policy discussions, especially in the areas of public education, science, and civil liberties, presuppose the legitimacy of political liberalism. This presupposition impedes the ability of proponents of the biblical worldview from shaping and influencing their culture and communities through public institutions. If political liberalism's claim to neutrality is difficult if not impossible to maintain,[17] then there is no reason in principle why Christian citizens

14. Rawls, *Political Liberalism*, p. xxviii.

15. Rawls, *Political Liberalism*, p. 10.

16. See, for example, Finnis, "Public Reason, Abortion, and Cloning;" Lee, *Abortion and Unborn Human Life;* John A. Mitchell and Scott B. Rae, "The Moral Status of Fetuses and Embryos," in *The Silent Subject: Reflections on the Unborn in American Culture,* ed. Brad Stetson (Westport, Conn.: Greenwood, 1996); Robert P. George and Gerard V. Bradley, "Marriage and the Liberal Imagination," *Georgetown Law Journal* 84 (1995); David Orgon Coolidge, *Same Sex Marriage?,* Crossroads Monograph Series in Faith and Public Policy, vol. 9 (Wynnewood, Pa.: Crossroads, 1996); and Nigel M. de S. Cameron, *The New Medicine: Life and Death After Hippocrates* (Wheaton, Ill.: Crossway Books, 1991).

17. For more thorough critiques of liberalism's apparent neutrality, see Francis Canavan, "The Pluralist Game" and "Liberalism in Root and Flower," in his *The Pluralist*

should not be able to employ the resources of liberal democracy to the same extent as their opposition.

A. Public Education and Political Liberalism

Let us consider *values clarification*. Made popular in the 1960s and 1970s, it has been used in many schools across America. It "is not concerned with the content of people's values, but the process of valuing." This approach ". . . does not teach a particular set of values. There is no sermonizing or moralizing. The goal is to involve the students in practical experiences, making them aware of their own feelings, their own ideas, their own beliefs, so that the choices and decisions they make are conscious and deliberate, based on their own value systems."[18]

Because values clarification is presented as a "neutral" theory that takes no position on what moral views are correct, opponents are often portrayed as narrow-minded moralists trying to force their views on others. Despite this portrayal, values clarification is really a partisan theory that affirms that there is only one correct morality, and that is personal subjective relativism: the view that there is no objective right and wrong that applies to all persons, in all times, and in all places. The embracing of relativism is clearly seen in the way in which the use of values clarification in the classroom dogmatically cuts off the search for truth, the primary purpose of education. To illustrate this, consider this dialogue (based loosely on a real-life exchange) between a high-school teacher and her student Elizabeth:

> **Teacher:** Welcome, students. This is the first day of class, and so I want to lay down some ground rules. First, since no one has the truth on religion and morality, you should be open-minded to the opinions of your fellow students. Second . . . Elizabeth, do you have a question?
>
> **Elizabeth:** Yes I do. If nobody has the truth, isn't that a good reason for me not to listen to my fellow students? After all, if nobody has the truth,

---

Game (Lanham, Md.: Rowman & Littlefield, 1995); George, "Public Reason and Political Conflict;" Sher, *Beyond Neutrality;* and Francis J. Beckwith and Gregory Koukl, *Relativism: Feet Firmly Planted in Mid-Air* (Grand Rapids: Baker, 1998).

18. S. B. Simon, L. W. Howe, and H. Kirschenbaum, *Values Clarification*, rev. ed. (New York: Hart, 1978), back cover; see also pp. 18-22. Quoted in Paul Vitz, "Why Values Clarification Must Be Rejected," *Do the Right Thing: A Philosophical Dialogue on the Moral and Social Issues of our Time,* ed. Francis J. Beckwith (Belmont, Calif.: Wadsworth, 1996), p. 83.

why should I waste my time listening to other people and their opinions? Only if somebody has the truth does it make sense to be open-minded. Don't you agree?

Teacher: No, I don't. Are you claiming to know the truth? Isn't that a bit arrogant and dogmatic?

Elizabeth: Not at all. Rather I think it's dogmatic, as well as arrogant, to assert that no single person on earth knows the truth. After all, have you met every person in the world and quizzed them exhaustively? If not, how can you make such a claim? Also, I believe it is actually the opposite of arrogance to say that I will alter my opinions to fit the truth whenever and wherever I find it. And if I happen to think that I have good reason to believe I do know the truth and would like to share it with you, why wouldn't you listen to me? Why would you automatically discredit my opinion before it is even uttered? I thought we were supposed to listen to everyone's opinion.

Teacher: This should prove to be an interesting semester.

Another Student (blurts out): Ain't that the truth. (The students laugh)[19]

The conflict over sex education is instructive here. Some parents and teachers are sometimes accused of promoting a religious agenda because they support abstinence education and oppose morally "neutral" sex education programs that teach among other things that homosexuality and sex outside of marriage are not inherently wrong because they are matters of individual choice.[20] These programs are in effect telling students that personal desire is

---

19. This dialogue is reproduced from Beckwith and Koukl, *Relativism,* p. 74.

20. Consider the American Civil Liberties Union's opposition to a 1988 California State Assembly bill, which mandated that abstinence be taught in sex education classes in public schools. In a letter written to the Assembly Education Committee (May 26, 1988), ACLU attorneys Marjorie C. Swartz and Francisco Lobaco argued that it is the ACLU's position "that teaching that monogamous heterosexual intercourse within marriage is a traditional American value is an unconstitutional establishment of a religious doctrine in public schools. There are various religions which hold contrary beliefs with respect to marriage and monogamy." (Reproduced in James Dobson and Gary L. Bauer, *Children at Risk* [Dallas: Word Publishing, 1990], p. 26.) Since one can be an atheist and agree with the assembly bill, it seems ludicrous for the ACLU to assert that the bill advances a religious doctrine. If the ACLU's position were to become official state policy, it is not difficult to believe that a teacher could be legally forbidden from telling Johnny that it is morally wrong to steal from Suzie, since the teacher's moral condemnation may be informed by her commitment to the truth of the Ten Commandments. In addition,

the primary arbiter when making judgments on the moral requirements of human sexuality. This assumes, however, a subjective and permissive view of sexuality, hardly a neutral one. By reducing sexuality to one's preferences, these programs are teaching students that human sexuality has no intrinsic purpose, and that certain social institutions, such as traditional marriage, are not normative. After all, if the authors of such curricula actually thought that their relativist view of sexuality could be wrong, or if they knew that a non-relativistic alternative were at least philosophically possible, they would not have ruled out, in principle, the possibility of ever having its discovery reflected in their curricula.

B. The Intelligent Design Movement

The above analysis can be applied to some of the concerns raised by the Intelligent Design Movement (IDM), a loosely connected group of academics in both Christian and secular institutions that is challenging naturalistic evolution by offering an alternative explanation of origins, an Intelligent Designer.[21] Although IDM raises many objections against *naturalistic evolution,* one is important for our discussion: naturalistic evolution assumes methodological naturalism, the view that affirms religious "neutrality" on the question of origins by requiring that the scientist, in order to practice science correctly, presuppose there is no Intelligent Designer or Creator.[22] The assumption of methodological naturalism is why courts have consistently rejected as unconstitutional legislation that requires that public schools teach creation if evolution is taught. These courts have maintained

---

teaching that the parameters of appropriate sexual behavior are limited only by personal choice, desire, and mutual consent — the view that the ACLU wants to be embodied in school curricula — is to further a view of human sexuality and family life grounded in the metaphysics of nominalism (the view that there are no designed natures or purposes in creation), which would put the state in the position of institutionalizing a partisan philosophical perspective. See Canavan, "The Pluralist Game" and "Liberalism in Root and Flower."

21. See, for example, William Dembski, ed., *Mere Creation* (Downers Grove, Ill.: InterVarsity, 1999); William Dembski, *The Design Inference* (New York: Cambridge University Press, 1998); and J. P. Moreland, ed., *The Creation Hypothesis* (Downers Grove, Ill.: InterVarsity, 1994).

22. See J. P. Moreland, "Theistic Science and Methodological Naturalism," in *The Creation Hypothesis;* and Phillip Johnson, *Reason in the Balance: The Case Against Naturalism in Science, Law, and Education* (Downers Grove, Ill.: InterVarsity Press, 1995), especially the appendix, "Naturalism, Methodological and Otherwise."

that teaching creation is teaching "religion" while teaching "evolution" is teaching science.[23]

Phillip Johnson, J. P. Moreland, and others point out, however, that methodological naturalism loads the dice so that any view, like intelligent design, that does not assume naturalism, is automatically rejected. Naturalism is a philosophical, not scientific, perspective that maintains that all that exists is the material world, that non-natural things like God, angels, souls, or morality do not actually exist. This means that any evidence or philosophical argument one may marshal for intelligent design, in the mind of the naturalist, does not matter, because God cannot be part of any scientific theory or even a leading character in the story of the universe's history. But this automatically excludes the theist from academic discourse that may challenge the primacy of naturalism, unless the theist is willing to capitulate and compartmentalize his metaphysical commitment. In other words, the theist has a right to believe in God but he dare not think that this belief is real knowledge that may also result from his cosmological reflections. This exclusion, however, is not the result of the naturalist having better arguments. Rather, it is the result of the naturalist and the naturalist's allies presupposing the truth of naturalism, and using the power structures of the most influential and culture-shaping institutions to marginalize or silence those who either harbor doubts about the status of naturalism as an epistemological starting point or think it wise to remove naturalism from its metaphysical throne. This is intellectual imperialism. It is not neutral.

Just as political liberalism, when embraced by the state, does not lead to state neutrality when it comes to policy issues that touch on normative questions of morality and sexuality, methodological naturalism, when embraced by the scientific community, does not lead to neutrality when it comes to philosophical questions that touch on the existence of an Intelligent Designer.

23. See *Edwards v. Aguillard* 482 U.S. 578 (1987) and *McLean v. Arkansas Board of Education* 1529 F.Supp. 1255 (W.D. Ark. 1982). For analyses of the reasoning in these decisions, see Stephen J. Gould, "Justice Scalia's Misunderstanding," *Constitutional Commentary* 5 (1988); Phillip E. Johnson, *Darwin on Trial* (Downers Grove, Ill.: InterVarsity Press, 1997), pp. 3-14, 111-22, 155-58; Johnson, *Reason in the Balance*, pp. 19-34, 220; Norman L. Geisler, A. F. Brooke, and Mark J. Keough, *The Creator in the Courtroom, "Scopes II": The Controversial Arkansas Creation-Evolution Trial* (Milford, Mich.: Mott Media, 1982); Larry Laudan, "Commentary: Science at the Bar — Causes for Concern," *Science, Technology, and Human Values* 7 (Fall 1982); J. P. Moreland, *Christianity and the Nature of Science* (Grand Rapids: Baker, 1989), pp. 213-46; and Francis J. Beckwith, "Are Creationists Philosophically and Scientifically Justified in Postulating God? A Critical Analysis of Naturalistic Evolution," *Interchange* 46 (1989).

C. Civil Liberties and Public Morality

Two moral issues that concern evangelicals are abortion and the proliferation of pornography, both of which are practices inconsistent with the biblical worldview.[24] Those who take a liberal stance on these issues typically maintain that a certain view of individual liberty (presumed as prima facie correct) justifies the state's permissive posture on these issues.

(1) *Abortion and State Neutrality.* Supporters of abortion rights typically argue for their position by appealing to state neutrality when it comes to matters of deeply held beliefs about the meaning and nature of life. They argue that the pro-choice position is neutral while the pro-life position is partisan because its proponents are trying to force their disputed moral views on others. Because of this, the pro-life position is intolerant and contrary to the American tradition of pluralism. The Supreme Court has provided us with two eloquent judgments that present reasons for this viewpoint. The first is from Justice Harry Blackmun's majority opinion in *Roe v. Wade* (1973): "We need not resolve the difficult question of when life begins. When those trained in the respective disciplines of medicine, philosophy, and theology are unable to arrive at any consensus, the judiciary, at this point in the development of man's knowledge, is not in a position to speculate."[25]

Blackmun's argument fails to establish government neutrality and thus the right to abortion,[26] for at least two reasons. First, the state, by leaving the choice of pregnancy termination solely to the discretion of pregnant women, is taking a definitive position on fetal personhood. It is affirming by its permission that the fetus is not worthy of state protection and therefore can be discarded without requiring any public justification whatsoever. Whatever one may think of this public policy, it is certainly not a neutral one. Although verbally the court denied taking sides, the practical effect of its opinion is that the fetus in this society is not a human person worthy of protection.

Imagine you are back in the nineteenth century and the court is confronted with the issue of enslaving African-Americans. Suppose, in the name of state neutrality, it delivers the opinion that it takes no stand on the issue. On that basis it *allows* white Americans to own blacks as property. It would appear that although the court is making a verbal denial of taking any position on this

---

24. I have, however, argued in my book *Politically Correct Death* that abortion to save the life of the mother is morally justified, for it is better that one should live than that two should perish.

25. *Roe v. Wade* 410 U.S. at 159.

26. For a detailed critique of this argument, see Francis J. Beckwith, "Ignorance of Fetal Personhood as a Justification of Abortion: A Critical Analysis," in *The Silent Subject.*

issue, the allowance of slavery is for all intents and purposes morally equivalent to taking a side on the issue, namely, that blacks are not human persons. Likewise, the court's verbal denial of taking a position on fetal personhood is contradicted by its conclusion that abortion is a fundamental constitutional right and that fetuses are not persons under the Constitution.[27]

Second, if we are to accept the Supreme Court's holding in *Roe*, and agree with Justice Blackmun that the right to abortion is contingent upon the status of the fetus,[28] then the allegedly disputed fact about life's beginning means that the right to abortion is disputed as well. For a conclusion's support — in this case, "abortion is a fundamental right" — is only as good as the veracity of its most important premise — in this case, "the fetus is not a human person." So, the court's admission that abortion-rights is based on a widely disputed fact, far from establishing a right to abortion, entails that the court not only does not know when life begins, but it does not know when, if ever, the right to abortion begins.

In *Casey v. Planned Parenthood* (1992), the court gives us another eloquent reason for state neutrality by asserting the primacy of personal autonomy over the metaphysical question of personhood:

> Our law affords constitutional protection to personal decisions relating to marriage, procreation, family relationships, child rearing, and education. . . . These matters, involving the most intimate and personal choices a person may make in a lifetime, choices central to personal dignity and autonomy, are central to the liberty protected by the Fourteenth Amendment. At the heart of liberty is the right to define one's own concept of existence, of meaning, of the universe, and of the mystery of human life. Beliefs about these matters could not define the attributes of personhood were they formed under compulsion by the State.[29]

27. Concerning the legal status of abortion in the United States, see the editors' introductory comments as well as the essays in part II of Louis P. Pojman and Francis J. Beckwith, eds., *The Abortion Controversy 25 Years After Roe v. Wade: A Reader*, 2nd ed. (Belmont, Calif.: Wadsworth, 1998).

28. Blackmun writes: "The appellee and certain amici argue that the fetus is a 'person' within the language and meaning of the Fourteenth Amendment. In support of this, they outline at length and in detail the well-known facts of fetal development. If this suggestion of personhood is established, the appellant's case, of course, collapses, for the fetus's right to life would then be guaranteed specifically by the Amendment. The appellant conceded as much on reargument. On the other hand, the appellee conceded on reargument that no case could be cited that holds that a fetus is a person within the meaning of the Fourteenth Amendment" (*Roe v. Wade* 410 U.S. at 157-58).

29. *Planned Parenthood v. Casey*, 112 Sup. Ct. 2807 (1992).

This is referred to by some as "the mystery passage."[30] Although much more can be said about this passage,[31] the following brief comments should suffice.

First, the proponents of the mystery passage presuppose the non-existence of an objective good or human nature. For if "the heart of liberty is the right to define one's own concept of existence, of meaning, of the universe, and of the mystery of human life," the court implies there is not a human good that one can know to be true, and thus, have reflected in our nation's legal framework. After all, if the court were not saying this, then it would have ruled in a way that would have implied or stated that knowing such a thing were at least philosophically possible. But the court's decision rules out the possibility of our legal framework ever having the discovery of an objective human good reflected in it.

Second, by upholding abortion rights in *Casey,* the court, as it did in *Roe,* defined the parameters of the human community by excluding certain human beings — fetuses — from protection by the state. Thus, even though it claims that "beliefs about these matters could not define the attributes of personhood were they formed under compulsion by the State," the court, an agent of the state, affirmed a particular view of personhood, which is, to say the least, controversial.

2. *Liberty and Obscenity.* The dominant view in contemporary jurisprudence maintains that "one has a prima facie obligation not to advocate or support any law or public policy that restricts human conduct, unless one has, and is willing to offer, adequate secular reason for this advocacy or support (say for one's vote)."[32] There is, in other words, a presumption in favor of "liberty." It is not clear, however, that this presumption has much explanatory power when it comes to the most controversial issues of our time, for this notion of liberty is part of a disputed framework of the social life against which one can raise reasonable counterexamples. If one can do that, then there is good reason to reject this presumption and thus reject this view of liberty as the default position. In order to make this point, let us consider a controversial issue from which we can derive counterexamples: censorship of obscenity and pornography.

---

30. I believe this description was coined by Notre Dame law professor Gerard V. Bradley in his article, "Shall We Ratify the New Constitution? The Judicial Manifesto in *Casey* and *Lee,*" in *Benchmarks: Great Constitutional Controversies in the Supreme Court,* ed. Terry Eastland (Washington, D.C.: Ethics & Public Policy Center/Grand Rapids: Eerdmans, 1995).

31. See, for example, Bradley, "Shall We Ratify the New Constitution?"

32. Audi, in *Religion in the Public Square,* p. 25.

Suppose that you are a parent who lives in a community in which pornography is widely distributed and easily accessible to adults.[33] It can be found with ease on the Internet, cable television (with outlets found in every home), and on the shelves of nearly every convenience store, movie rental business, and book retailer. In addition, radio-talk stations, which specialize in vulgar conversation, occasionally have guests from the adult film industry. Your children's friends and their parents sometimes listen to these programs when they drive together to work and school. While at home you tell your teenage sons that regular consumption of pornography is harmful to their souls; that it will give them a distorted view of women; and that this may have a negative effect upon intimacy in their future marriages. You point out, moreover, that since pornography appeals to the desires rather than to the intellect, it is not something that one can indulge in freely for very long, for one can become a slave to one's base desires. So, you tell your boys, "Even though I am forbidding you access to pornography, I am in reality giving you more freedom, for this restriction of your conduct will make it less likely that you will become a slave to your desires."

You quickly realize, however, that because of your community's unwillingness to create and nurture a climate in which access to pornography is regulated, it is next to impossible for you to adequately fulfill your parental duty (not to mention your duty as a citizen concerned with the moral ecology of your community). Your boys, moreover, begin to resent your protective restrictions, for they feel deprived of what other boys in your community have an easy opportunity to enjoy. Nevertheless, you live in a *libertine* community, a community that defines liberty as freedom to do whatever one pleases as long one does not interfere with another's liberty to do the same. Any restrictions on another's liberty, based on a disputed view of the good life, are prima facie wrong. At the same time you know that libertinism is disputed, and therefore, based on the very same doctrine of state neutrality used against legislating your perspective, ought not to have a privileged position in your community's legal and social framework. For it seems to you quite plain that your parental duty to raise your children in a way you judge appropriate is being severely hampered by someone else's "community standards." As Robert P. George points out:

> People, notably including children, are formed not only in households, but in neighborhoods, and wider communities. Parents can prohibit a

---

33. This illustration was inspired by a similar one given by Robert P. George in *Making Men Moral*, p. 27.

certain act, but their likelihood of success in enforcing the prohibition, and transmitting to their children a genuine grasp of the wrongness of the prohibited act, will be lessened to the extent that others more or less freely perform the act. . . .

Whatever authority parents have over their children, they lack the authority to deprive other people in the community, or other people's children, of the legal liberty to perform immoral acts; only public officials possess authority of that kind. If, however, public authorities fail to combat certain vices, the impact of widespread immorality on the community's moral environment is likely to make the task of parents to rightly forbid their own children from, say, indulging in pornography, extremely difficult.[34]

Thus, from your perspective, your community's liberty to enjoy pornography, and your government's unwillingness to do anything about it, restricts you and your freedom.

In addition, because you are firmly convinced that indulgence in pornography is the sort of activity that often results in the consumers becoming enslaved by their lusts, you also believe that this enslavement harms marriages and the children in those households. Those children, because of their upbringing, are likely not to become as well adjusted adults as those children brought up in more intact homes where pornography is not consumed. You know this from personal experience, philosophical reflection, as well as your religious tradition, which you believe is true and can be defended by rational arguments (broadly defined).

Ironically, as part of the defense of your position, you employ the "golden rule" application of libertinism: "[It] is a kind of restraint I would wish to be observed by members of other religious groups who would want to coerce my behavior in the direction of their religiously preferred standards."[35] You reason thusly: "Since I know that I have a weakness of will, and a propensity to do what is wrong if there are no legal barriers to discourage me, I am grateful when the state forbids a bad behavior. It liberates me from the call of temptation. Virtue is easier to attain when there is encouragement by members of the wider community, and that encouragement is reflected in the legal framework. Because I believe that the legal framework ought to make it difficult for me to treat myself in a degrading and immoral way, and I am grateful when it does, I owe it to my fellow citizens to help make it easier for them to live a virtuous life as well." In the words of John Finnis, your legis-

---

34. George, *Making Men Moral*, p. 27.
35. Audi, in *Religion in the Public Square*, p. 51.

lative proposal "*may* manifest, not contempt, but a sense of equal human worth of those people, whose conduct is outlawed precisely on the ground that it expresses a serious misconception of, and actually degrades, human worth and dignity, and thus degrades their own personal worth and dignity, along with that of others who may be induced to share in or emulate their degradation."[36] The fact that your notion of virtue is connected to a disputed comprehensive doctrine (or religious viewpoint) is irrelevant, for, as we have seen, libertinism, the alleged default position, is also based on a disputed comprehensive doctrine. Since the issue is whether the latter should be the default position, it is clear that it does not achieve that status because *your* position is disputed, for libertinism is equally contested.

Recall the principle on which libertinism is grounded: "[O]ne has a prima facie obligation not to advocate or support any law or public policy that restricts human conduct, unless one has, and is willing to offer, adequate secular reason for this advocacy or support (say for one's vote)."[37] In light of the above illustration, this principle seems to be an inadequate guide because it lacks explanatory power. After all, from your perspective, lack of censorship restricts human conduct because it disrupts the fragile moral community that is necessary for human flourishing and true liberty. But from the perspective of the connoisseur of pornography, your call for censorship is restricting his conduct. Because it is not clear from this example which view of freedom should have the presumption; and because most other "liberty" issues can be examined under the same analysis and lead to similar conclusions; there is no reason to suppose that this view of freedom should have the presumption. It seems, then, that citizens who embrace this view of freedom should not win by default, but should also have, and must be willing to offer, adequate reason for the viewpoints they advocate and support. After all, from *your* perspective, it is their policies that are restricting human conduct.

*   *   *

As long as Christians, and evangelicals in particular, continue to engage the culture within the parameters, and by the rules, authorized by their philosophical adversaries, the prospect of cultural change is bleak. This is why I have made a case for cultural engagement that is based on what has been

36. John Finnis, "Legal Enforcement of 'Duties to Oneself': Kant v. Neo-Kantians," *Columbia Law Review* 67 (1987): 437.
37. Audi, in *Religion in the Public Square*, p. 25.

called "worldview analysis."[38] Instead of *merely* looking at isolated issues, this approach challenges the philosophical presuppositions that are doing the intellectual work in the minds of those who reject the biblical worldview as a legitimate basis by which to ground our cultural framework. This approach successfully challenges the claim of secularists that their position is both neutral and not committed to any controversial philosophical positions on the good, the true, and the beautiful. For political liberalism's claim to neutrality masks its metaphysical and epistemological commitment to philosophical naturalism and views of morality, sexuality, origins, human personhood, and social thought that typically flow from that commitment.

38. See, for example, Ronald H. Nash, *Worldviews in Conflict* (Grand Rapids: Zondervan, 1992).

Biomedical Ethics and
U.S. Health Policy

Scott E. Daniels, Ph.D.

Introduction

The United States government's attempt over the past three decades to fashion an ethical consensus on biomedical advances amid a pluralistic society has generally led to establishing federal bioethics commissions. During the mid-to-late 1960s, public concern regarding the treatment of human beings in biomedical research gave rise in the 1970s to the National Commission for the Protection of Human Subjects of Biomedical and Behavioral Research. Most of the recommendations from this commission have become the current regulatory structure for protecting humans in a variety of research contexts codified as 45 Code of Federal Regulation 46. Social apprehension about applying breakthrough biotechnologies in the delivery of health care resulted in the early 1980s in the creation of the President's Commission for the Study of Ethical Problems in Medicine and Biomedical and Behavioral Research. These two bodies are the most well known federal ethics initiatives. But their tenure was not permanent.

One of the regulations protecting human subjects adopted during the 1970s required that the secretary of the Department of Health and Human Services appoint an Ethics Advisory Board (EAB) to review research involving in vitro embryos and determine whether the project was ethically acceptable. Without the EAB's review, this type of research could not be approved for federal funding. The EAB had convened only once for a fleeting period during 1978 to 1980 to review research regarding in vitro fertilization (IVF).

Proponents of embryo research argued that the absence of the EAB since 1980 served as a *de facto* moratorium on funding in vitro embryo research.

Congress established a congressional Biomedical Ethics Committee in 1985 to address these sensitive issues as a way of partly circumventing the Health and Human Services regulation. But membership selection eventually killed the committee before it could issue a single report. Since the 1980s, there have been several *ad hoc* ethics panels. With the notable exception of the independent panel on Human Fetal Tissue Transplantation Research, most of these entities have been obscure. This chapter is a review of the controversial history of these ethical bodies from a personal perspective. During the heated debate over the use of fetal tissue for transplantation, I was a political appointee in the Office of the Assistant Secretary of Health, as well as a professional staffer for Senator Orrin G. Hatch on the Committee on Labor and Human Resources, given the task of managing this high profile issue. I will survey the federal initiatives in the realm of biomedical ethics and public policy. I also will give an overview of the types of federal initiatives, survey the topics addressed, and critique the ethical perspectives from which these analyses were carried out. I shall raise ethical objections to the utility of this *nationalized* way of doing bioethics. Then, we will do a little reflective thinking ourselves and ask, what is the role of theology in bioethical public policy?

Historical Setting Leading to the National Commissions

We are all familiar with the atrocities committed by physicians in Nazi concentration camps during World War II. This period marked a new phase in the history of bioethics. Other horrifying events in the United States are less well known. Several historic examples of abuses may be mentioned from the 1950s, 1960s, and 1970s. Tuskegee brings to mind the unethical nontreatment of syphilis among African-Americans in Alabama. The Brooklyn Chronic Disease Hospital case involved injecting live cancer cells into unconsenting elderly patients. The Willowbrook incident involved the use of incarcerated, mentally retarded children to test hepatitis vaccines. And there are anecdotal reports of improper use of fetuses in biomedical research in the early 1970s at the National Institutes of Health (NIH) or at institutions supported by the NIH. As a marginal note, news accounts earlier in this decade reported that the federal government inappropriately exposed unsuspecting Americans to doses of radiation earlier in this century as a means of studying the effects of a nuclear attack.

As a result of this cascade of unethical events, the United States has been engaged in substantial biomedical ethical debate for more than three decades. These discussions have been carried out within the formal structure of national ethics commissions or panels. With few exceptions, evangelicals have rarely been invited to participate as members of these bodies. Nevertheless, these bioethical debates are of concern to evangelicals. Questions such as whether, and under what circumstances, it is permissible to conduct nontherapeutic investigations on fetuses; to manipulate human genes; to withhold medical treatment; and to allocate finite medical resources are issues that cut to the core of God's created order.

The Federal Initiatives in Biomedical Ethics Public Policy

Government efforts to enter the realm of biomedical ethics have been, and continue to be, highly controversial. The success of these initiatives also continues to be a matter of debate. There have been several failed attempts to establish a body whose rulings would centralize ethical guidelines. Proponents of federal ethical initiatives see them as granting permission to engage in research activities that the larger social ethos finds abhorrent. (If not unrestricted permission, the authorization for investigations under an elaborate set of provisos.) In the instances where limits have been imposed on science, the biomedical and medical community has strongly resisted them as unwarranted concessions to an unenlightened society — even if it has temporarily tolerated these prohibitions. Such is the case of restricting research that poses more than minimal risk to the fetus without therapeutic benefit for the fetus.

Opponents of federal efforts to centralize biomedical ethical decision-making generally see the government's refusal to set serious limits on certain research activities as attempts to use the benevolence of medical research as a tool to forge larger social transformation in moral thinking.

The National Commission for the Protection of Human Subjects of Biomedical and Behavioral Research (known as National Commission) was created in July 1974 and completed its last report in 1978. Its mission was "to identify the basic ethical principles which should underlie the conduct of biomedical and behavioral research involving human subjects." It was also to make recommendations regarding federal implementation of these principles in government research. Its eleven-member panel was appointed by the Secretary of the Department of Health, Education, and Welfare (forerunner to the Department of Health and Human Services). The membership included five scientists, three lawyers, two ethicists, and one person in public affairs.

The National Commission issued eleven reports. These reports included ethical guidelines to protect classes of vulnerable human subjects — presumably as a response to the abuses mentioned in the introductory remarks — such as fetuses, prisoners, children, and the mentally infirm. The commission also issued reports on research conducted as part of delivering health care and psychosurgery. Moreover, it made recommendations for the inclusion of ethical guidelines in the review processes of the institutional review boards (IRBs), which exist in all major U.S. research centers. Finally, *the Belmont Report,* its most celebrated issuance, which analyzed the ethical principles, became the basis of ethical analysis for future commissions and panels, and the IRBs. Within a short period, the Department of Health, Education, and Welfare converted the National Commission's recommendation into regulations (known as 45 Code of Federal Regulation 46).

In compliance with the National Commission's recommendations, President Jimmy Carter's secretary of Health, Education, and Welfare convened the first Ethics Advisory Board (EAB). The mission of the EAB was less sweeping than that of the National Commission (and of the President's Commission, which we will be reviewing next), and it was tied to a review of actual research projects. Its task was to advise the secretary on the "acceptability from an ethical standpoint" of specific research protocols. It, too, was an eleven-member board with similar membership composition. Although it was intended to be a permanently standing body with jurisdiction over research conducted with the Department of Health and Human Services, controversy surrounding its key ruling contributed to its termination in 1980 after two years.

During this two-year interval, the EAB issued a very controversial report on in vitro fertilization and embryo transfer. One of the EAB's central conclusions was that IVF was acceptable from the ethical standpoint. It was careful, however, to point out that this standard did not mean "clearly ethically right," but "ethically defensible but still legitimately controverted." The EAB determined that IVF research *without* embryo transfer was acceptable from an ethical standpoint. The EAB presented qualifications with their approval. One, the research must advance the scientific understanding of the safety and efficacy of embryo transfer. Two, the knowledge gained through the research could not be reasonably attainable by other means. Third, no embryo would be sustained beyond fourteen days after fertilization. The EAB also concluded that IVF research with embryo transfer is acceptable as long as the gametes are taken from married couples, and the embryo is transferred back into the wife whose ova were used for fertilization.

The EAB was not reconvened after 1980. This has led some proponents of controversial research to charge that there was a *de facto* moratorium on this category of research, and that Health and Human Services stands in violation of its own regulations.

The President's Commission for the Study of Ethical Problems in Medicine and Biomedical and Behavioral Research (known as the President's Commission) replaced the EAB in the early 1980s. Secretary Joseph A. Califano Jr. redirected funding from the EAB to the newly established President's Commission. Critics often alleged that the Department of Health, Education, and Welfare misunderstood the differing purposes of the two ethical bodies. The EAB reviewed specific research projects while the President's Commission focused on the broader philosophical aspects of biomedical ethics policy. The EAB admittedly was given the task of reviewing actual protocol applications. But its scope was not necessarily limited to such specificity. Testimony delivered to the Subcommittee on Health and the Environment House Committee on Interstate and Foreign Commerce on August 4, 1978, suggests that Califano revised the EAB's charter to be broader in scope. The concurrent existence of the two bodies would have meant significant overlap in mission — with the President's Commission having greater authority. The two bodies were for practical reasons unnecessary.

The President's Commission was an eleven-member, rotating panel with six members being appointed from medicine and biomedical research. The topics focused principally on the practical application of biomedical research. During its three-year tenure, it released sixteen volumes covering subjects like informed consent, decisions to forgo life-sustaining treatment, definition of death, access to health care, genetic screening and counseling, genetic engineering, compensation for injury from biomedical research, and IRB regulation.

President Reagan refused to reappoint members to the President's Commission in 1983. So, in 1985 then-Senator Al Gore successfully pushed legislation establishing the Congressional Biomedical Ethics Advisory Committee. This panel was from the very beginning plagued by the politics of membership. There was fervent battling between those in Congress who attached significance to the sanctity of life and those who did not. The controversy was over control of the fourteen-member committee. But the fierce effort manifested itself when one of the five appointed "pro-life" members died. When a compromise on the selection of a new member was finally struck, media reports indicated that the newly appointed executive director made inappropriate public statements to the effect that the abortion supporters had prevailed in gaining stronger representation, and hence a majority on the commission. The perspective of the executive director, moreover, disclosed the potential orientation of the selection of commission staff, who would control the research and drafting of recommendations. The panel was promptly killed by "pro-life" senators who had suffered embarrassment at the defeat of the pro-life issue.

The Biomedical Ethics Advisory Committee disbanded before it could issue a single report. But the statutory topics mandated by Congress included human genetic engineering (gene therapy), fetal research, and nutrition and hydration of dying patients.

There have been several other attempts at federal intervention into biomedical ethical public policy-making. Most of these efforts were *ad hoc* panels with short tenures. The most celebrated was the Human Fetal Tissue Transplantation Research Panel. Likewise, this panel was sullied by controversies surrounding abortion and other issues. Only three slots on the twenty-one-member panel were occupied by individuals who resisted the apparent pro-research leaning of the panel. Their dissenting minority report reversed the long-standing trend of consensus and unanimity in decision-making characteristic of previous commissions.

During the 1990s two significant developments occurred. First, in 1993 federal legislation was enacted reauthorizing the funds supporting the National Institutes for Health repealing the controversial regulation requiring EAB approval for embryo research. Research on in vitro embryos set off a new round of controversy. In 1994, President Clinton signed an Executive Order, which among other things, created a National Ethics Advisory Commission. The commission has sweeping authority and is currently deliberating over research on the use of stem cells taken from in vitro embryos.

The Ethical Perspective of the Federal Commissions

A most telling summary of the perspective underlying the federal bioethics commissions, boards, and panels is found in a report, *Biomedical Ethics in U.S. Public Policy* (June 1993) produced by the U.S. Congressional Office of Technology Assessment (OTA).[1] This study presented the insights of most of the previous participants of the various federal initiatives. All, without exception, were proponents of a centralized control of biomedical ethical guidelines, though there were disagreements as to the form and structure of such a body. It came as no surprise that the critical perspective advocated in the report was a capitulation to our contemporary moral confusion.

1. The Office of Technology Assessment was a branch of the U.S. Congress. It was eliminated in the mid-1990s.

In the absence of a single authoritarian church or other mechanisms to handle bioethical issues, American society often turns to government or the courts for resolution of thorny ethical issues. The reemerging interest in the role of bioethics in U.S. public policy signals the increasing importance of medical and biological technologies in daily life. The creation of federal commissions stems from a desire for mechanisms to articulate common values and foster consensus in the face of growing cultural and religious heterogeneity. (p. 7)

As to the report's assessment of our ethical plight, it reiterated the characteristic pragmatic doctrine: "The need is not so much for finding moral solutions to complex policy matters, but rather, for identifying problems and either making recommendations or defining tradeoffs among alternatives" (p. 7).

The significance that OTA and its conferees attached to this state of affairs is quite unclear. It is uncertain whether they found this moral breakdown a collapse of an obsolete tradition with the confusion attending the emergence of an enlightened alternative, or an inevitable — and desirable — expression of a pluralistic society. Perhaps, though I doubt it, they were lamenting the loss of a solid tradition and seeking ways to reestablish it.

It is clear, however, that the federal commissions are viewed as a necessary "mechanism" to guide us through a period of time in which biomedical advances apparently outpace ethical judgment. Those touchstone values on which these initiatives must rely are the same as those developed as part of the National Commission's analyses. These include autonomy, beneficence, and justice. Upon these ethical principles, the panels have attempted to forge a consensus and impose this consensus upon the whole of society. In this regard, the OTA report is at pains to justify the influence that the studies and papers have had on education curriculum, court rulings, medical practices, and the like. Indeed, these are the marks of "success" it attributes to the commissions. Today over 250 research centers across the United States conduct ethical reviews using the ethical principles presented by the 1970s National Commission.

Less obvious and largely presumed is an implicit commitment to the scientific imperative. The scientific imperative attaches importance to a single value, to advancing research without regard to content of the research project. This is reflected in several ways. Not least, the panels are composed largely of clinical and medical researchers. More importantly, however, the principle of beneficence is usually presented as a general scientific goal of serving an obvious humanitarian good (for instance, alleviating human suffering or helping infertile couples bear children). Consequently, moral considerations about the larger social impact of the means to achieving that end (such as terminating innocent human life) are devalued by comparison. In fact, concerns about abortion are neutralized by reference to its legality. The intellectual integrity of individuals with commitments to the sanctity of life is automatically suspect and jeopardizes their opportunity to serve on the commission as a member. As the OTA report puts it: "Ideology is a destructive criterion in appointing a bioethics committee" (p. 34).

Thus, unanimity and consensus, another implicit procedural value, are threatened. This certainly was the case in the Human Fetal Tissue Transplantation Panel, which under great pressure finally — and reluctantly — published a minority opinion from the three dissenters (out of twenty-one panelists). But even then, the minority report was tempered by the chairman's decision to publish a rebuttal separate from the majority report. Although consensus has a distinctive advantage of busting through cultural barriers to create a new consciousness, it has serious problems of generating an impoverished morality unable to make fine distinctions in complex situations. It reduces the aim of morality to seeking subjective agreements, rather than pursuing moral truth. Finally, it inevitably eliminates challenging and prophetic viewpoints.

The moral prophets may indeed be those who defend the traditional conscience by exposing the excesses of moral self-expressivism. In short, society is ill-served by imposing on it a morality with the lowest common denominator. It surely is open to question whether this new moral point of view is any better than our traditional moorings in managing the rapid increase of biomedical advances. For that matter, it may be that the paradoxes we ascribe to scientific advance have more to do with the impoverishment of the emerging contemporary ethical perspective than with technological applications themselves.

One obvious instance of the impoverished nature of the scheme is its exclusion of respect for human life. The value is presumed in research, but never given explicit credit. For example, gene therapy aims to minimize suffering. But in many cases where the technology might be applied, the logical conclusion from this single-valued perspective should be to let the patient die. Yet, no biomedical researcher would suggest such an option. By contrast, I would argue that the aim of minimizing suffering is understood in the context of respect for human life as the bearer of experience. It is this more fundamental intuition that accounts for the urgency attributed to alleviating suffering through this biotechnology.

Moreover, the "enlightened" scheme involving only beneficence, justice, and autonomy is incoherent. The principles are undefined. Space does not permit illustration of this in detail, but the best instance I am aware of was the debate several years ago concerning whether the U.S. Health Care Financing Administration should waive federal requirements so that Oregon could ration care to its Medicaid population. I remember being asked to write a memo on whether or not the IRB regulation would lead to a satisfactory solution. My view was that no solution could be found. Why? The principle of justice was left undefined. Accordingly, when applying even a liberal theory of justice, like that of John Rawls,[2] the result led to contradictory conclusions. The crux of the problem was the question, "What is the basic demand of justice in Rawls's system?" Does it entail the stringent requirement of "not making anyone worse off" or "making the poor better off"? The regulations give no guidance here. As academic as this sounds, it was a real issue with ultra-liberals coming down on both sides of the question. Representatives Ron Wyden and Henry Waxman defended the Oregon plan while Gore called it "unfair." These political figures made their case on the basis of justice.

The "enlightened" scheme is incoherent in yet a second way. The commissions have not provided any method for deciding conflicts between these ethical principles (beneficence, autonomy, and justice). Even today the federal regulation provides no guidance on this basic theoretical demand. The researcher's compliance involves nothing more than saying something about how these three values apply to his research project. Likewise, the IRB is in no better position to evaluate the merits of researchers' projects. Thus, the process through which the regulatory demands are met regarding the ethical concerns is tantamount to muddling through.

Finally, there is the problem of impugning the integrity of biomedical ethics. The "sociological" approach of constituting the multidisciplinary panels of professionals invites politicization of the panels' rulings from all sides. After all, these centralized pronouncements will ultimately affect the health-care system for which citizens pay taxes and by which they are served. If the ordinary person can anticipate that the final outcome of a commission's deliberations will be to merely sanction a pro-research agenda (albeit a sophisticated and subtle form of the ends-justifies-the means) based on the scientific membership of the panel, the public will readily become cynical toward this "mechanism for articulating common values." Thus, the enterprise of biomedical ethics is ultimately undermined. Ethics is nothing without voluntary allegiance. The commissions' findings will never be able to gain the allegiance of ordinary people. To many a layperson the rulings appear as nothing more

2. John Rawls, *A Theory of Justice* (Cambridge, Mass.: The Belknap Press of Harvard University Press, 1971).

than political sophistry. Thus, the integrity of biomedical ethics rulings is damaged beyond repair.

The Christian Stake in Bioethics

What role does theology have in the biomedical ethics debate — particularly that part of it that affects public policy? In addressing this question, the believer immediately confronts a dilemma. Either the principles that apply to medical practice and research are discernible to reasonable persons, or religion provides merely one among many alternatives in a pluralistic society from which to view moral issues. In the first instance, theology is irrelevant; in the second, it is intrusive — especially because pluralism removes the urge to show that one view is preferable to another. Of course, because pluralism has become the very air we breathe in the United States, this argument against believers' involvement confronts yet another obstacle, which is simply to press for the highest degree of consensus possible.

One of our most powerful human intuitions is that moral judgments are not created by choice. In short, morality is — to use J. L. Mackie's pejorative phrase — "required by the universe."[3] And, this intuition is something we share with the human community. That is, as a matter of creation in God's image, the Creator has made our moral intuitions *trustworthy*, though not infallible.

So, part of the Christian stake in bioethics is to show this dilemma to be false. I think that a case against this dilemma should follow these general contours. The case should show that Christian theology is relevant because it enriches our understanding of ethical principles by offering coherent explanations for our moral intuitions. A second part of this case will be to recognize that moral values make reference to human nature. Nature here means God's ordained, humanly significant purposes. Human nature is in this sense not identical to physiological processes, even though physiological processes typically promote and express these purposes.

To pursue this route captures the genuine goal of bioethics, which is setting limits in accord with the ordained human purpose, rather than granting permission to proceed — albeit with all proper cautionary warnings. The ordinary conscience more than the trained mind of the biomedical researcher, with all its best intentions, is particularly keen to this distinction.

Tempted by alluring research opportunities to "improve" our genetic

---

3. J. L. Mackie, *Ethics: Inventing Right and Wrong* (New York: Penguin, 1977).

endowment beyond ways that could charitably be called restoration, the ordinary person expresses his refusal to "play God." Leaving aside the familiar issues raised by abortion, the possibility of controlling the sex of a child, using fetal organs (such as ovaries or brain tissue) as implants, or exploring the frontiers of in vitro fertilization runs contrary to our natural piety to accept human life as a *gift;* something given and not to be manipulated. It is significant that these religious expressions remain so widely current. They capture the felt apprehensions of the ordinary person's ethical intuitions to set limits to human creations. By themselves, these residual intuitions lack sufficient explanation and justification. Neither the Kantian emphasis on the autonomous person — which arbitrarily bifurcates our rational and sensible selves — nor the utilitarian stress on consequences directed at maximizing or minimizing certain experiences (such as suffering), can adequately explain these commonsense inhibitions. Without a theological framework that provides them full explanation, they are susceptible to distortion by other intellectual forces. I think the ordinary conscience is right, and at the same time authentically Christian.

How the Law Will Shape
Our Life and Death Decisions:
The Case of the Human Embryo

Samuel B. Casey, J.D.

To my left, we have *Dr. Asclepius,* our currently proud, but sometimes befuddled, symbol for *Medicine,* holding his chart of inquiry and his test tube full of life. He rarely has time for Justice, but she just won't leave him alone. To my right, we have *Lady Justice,* our currently blinded symbol for the *Law,* holding her scales of equality (reflecting the dignity of all human beings before the law) and her sword of judgment for life or death. She occasionally uses her sword rather than her reason to find her way. She is not nearly as blind as people think or hope. She *is* attracted to Dr. Asclepius and has trouble leaving him alone. She so wants him to like her. He wants her to leave him alone. They have a problem.

Medicine and Law currently *do* have a problem. They do not agree when human life begins. They neither trust nor understand each other very well. Power and technology and fear throw them together all the time. Their practitioners are ever more frequently accused of the "M" word (malpractice) by their patients or clients. Both are confused about their own identities and appropriate powers. Their problem is not new.

The older version of their story is Lady Justice only gave Asclepius a life-preserving vial, reserving the power of destruction for herself. "Why else," says Lady Justice, "do you think *I* am still carrying around *this* sword?" The more modern version of their story is that Lady Justice gave Asclepius, the revered founder of Medicine, *two* vials: one provided protection against death, and the other contained deadly poison. The potions are hard to tell apart. Lady Justice also lets Asclepius take her sword, as well, from time to time.

According to Dr. Leon Kass of the University of Chicago, "there is force to both accounts: the first shows that wisdom would constitute medicine an unqualifiedly benevolent — i.e. intrinsically ethical — art." The second attests to the moral neutrality of medical means, and of technical power generally;[1] Hippocrates — the inspiration for medicine's Hippocratic oath, still administered in more than 95 percent of our medical schools — favored the first version when he wrote in *The Epidemics:* "As to diseases, make a habit of two things — to help, or at least do no harm."[2]

Today, we doubt that medicine is an intrinsically ethical activity, but we are quite certain it can both help and harm. In fact, today help and harm flow from the same vial. The same respirator that brings a woman back from the edge of the grave also senselessly prolongs the life of an irreversibly comatose man. The same morphine that reverses the respiratory distress of pulmonary edema, in higher doses arrests respiration altogether. Whether they want to or not, doctors are able to kill — quickly, efficiently, and surely. And what is more, the law, particularly judge-made law, seems to be letting doctors kill more often and more openly. This is either to protect the autonomy (privacy) or "liberty" rights of their "patients" (in the cases of abortion and physician-assisted suicide), or to celebrate the allegedly humane and compassionate motives of the doctors or medical researchers (in the cases of abortion, euthanasia, in vitro fertilization, pre-implantation embryonic screening, or human embryonic stem cell research).

Law is not without *her* problems. Fifteen years ago John T. Noonan, the most respected pro-life legal scholar in America, published his justly famous essay, "The Root and Branch of Roe v. Wade."[3] Noonan, a Roman Catholic writing in the natural law tradition, found the "root" of *Roe* to be the positivist belief that the sovereign has an absolute right to define who counts as a person with rights. Under this positivist view, the law does not need to correspond to reality or nature; a human being could at will be relegated to the legal status of real estate, kitchen utensils, or livestock. Noonan noted that eminent lawyers such as Thomas Jefferson and Abraham Lincoln had engaged in these sorts of characterizations in relation to slavery law. The law, Noonan ar-

1. Dr. Leon R. Kass, "Neither for Love or Money: Why Doctors Must Not Kill," *The Human Life Review* 15 (1989): 93.

2. Hippocrates, *Epidemics 1, XI. Hippocrates, Volume 1*, trans. W. H. S. Jones (Cambridge, Mass.: Harvard University Press, 1964), p. 165.

3. Neb. L. Rev. 63 (1984): 668; see also David M. Smolin, "The Root and Branch of Anti-Abortion Lawlessness," *Baylor L. Rev.* 47 (1995): 119.

gued, became a "mask obliterating the human person." Noonan argued that *Roe* and its progeny had used the law as a mask to avoid perceiving "the reality of the extraordinary beauty of each human being put to death in the name of the abortion liberty." As we will see, the extraordinary and unique "beauty" of the human being, in his or her embryonic age, is now being put to death in the name of the "research" liberty.

Noonan described the "branch" of *Roe* as the Supreme Court's invention of doctrine unconstrained by the text or purposes of the Constitution. Noonan called such doctrine — the abortion right — "fantasy in the service of ideology." This branch was a reflection of the positivist logic which, in Noonan's words, "permits the judges at the apex of a system to dispense with correspondence to reality."[4] The positivist root permitted the justices to declare human beings "non-persons"; the positivist branch permitted the justices to invent constitutional doctrines without regard to the Constitution. In both instances, positivism gave justices the right to shape law with no correspondence to reality.

Insofar as the declaration of the abortion right also patently contravenes the will of the people, as expressed in the legislative enactments of the several states nullified by *Roe* and the rulings that followed, such legal positivism has also been critically referred to more recently as the *"judicial usurpation of democracy."*[5]

Noonan believed that natural law, properly understood and applied, could serve to prevent the evils created by positivism's absolutist view of state power. A decade later, however, it has been suggested that the natural law–based absolutisms of the anti-abortion movement have led to the recent murders of physicians and others involved in the provision of abortion services. There is no doubt that Noonan, and the overwhelming majority of those who share his views, condemn those killings. Nonetheless, it is not enough for those who believe in moral absolutes to condemn these murders, or to point

---

4. In reality, the question as to "when a human being begins is strictly a scientific question and should be answered by human embryologists — not philosophers, bioethicists, theologians, politicians, judges, x-ray technicians, movie stars or obstetricians and gynecologists. Current discussions on abortion, human embryo research (including cloning, stem cell research, and the formation of mixed species chimera) and the use of abortifacients involve specific claims as to when the life of every human being begins." Dianne N. Irving, Ph.D., "When Do Human Beings Begin? Scientific Myths and Scientific Facts" (on file with author).

5. See Richard John Neuhaus et al., *The End of Democracy? The Judicial Usurpation of Politics* (Spence Publishing, 1997); *The End of Democracy II: A Crisis of Legitimacy* (Spence Publishing, 1999).

out the obvious incongruities involved in killing in the name of life. The more profound questions concern the role that a claim of moral absolutes can and should play within legal and public debate. Noonan, and the natural law tradition he represents, warns of the dangers of absolutist tyranny posed by positivism; the countercharge is that claims based on natural law possess an absolutism that also can be dangerous.

Any answer to these questions must begin with the understanding that competing concepts of law, and hence lawlessness, are at the root of the life and death decisions confronting the law today. The concept of law we adopt will direct how the law shapes our views of the issues.

On the one hand, positivism finds lawfulness to stem from consent. The priority of the right (over the good) means that a system is legitimate if it grants moral autonomy to individuals; individuals have the right not to be coerced without their consent. Thus, particularistic religious and moral claims are not sufficient to legitimize either the political system as a whole, or particular legal rules, as both must be justified by "public reasons," or reasons accessible to all. Particularistic religious beliefs rely on claims of divine authority that are not shared by all persons, and hence some say it is "lawless" to use them in public political debate. God's "will," whatever it may be, has no more authority than that of any member of the political community; the political community, in that sense, protects the "right" of every human to deny God's authority. God, or those who would uphold God's authority within the political community, become "lawless" in this view. Consequently, to be heard and judged to be lawful by legal positivists, it is best to be able to cite "public reasons." Theoretically, one would think that the best "public reasons" would be a duly enacted statute. However, even duly enacted statutes are often held to be unconstitutional when they seek to define when a human being begins.

On the other hand, the natural law tradition finds human will, whether of each individual or even of a community, too arbitrary to constitute a foundation for either a political system, or even a particular law. Thus, Noonan is horrified at the positivist result that "there is no kind of human behavior that, because of its nature, could not be made into a legal duty corresponding to a legal right." The natural law tradition grounds all law in reason, which is understood as participating in the moral law of God as revealed in nature. The good precedes the right, and hence there is no "right" to choose evil, or to define that which is by nature evil, as good. A strictly positivistic system is thus, in a sense, a lawless system, particularly when its laws contradict the natural law. An unjust law is no law at all, regardless of the will of the individual or the community.

Judging how the law will shape our life and death decisions is complicated by these contrasting visions of lawfulness and lawlessness. Natural law and evangelical interpretations of "law" perceive *Roe* as lawless in several senses. *First,* Roe makes a seriously harmful act contrary to the higher law into a "right," and thus trumps both reason and good by the arbitrary will of each pregnant woman. *Second,* Roe itself is an arbitrary act of the Supreme Court justices which subverts the law of the "Constitution" through the arbitrary will of the justices, and hence makes all future law subject to the same subversion. *Third,* Roe fails even under positivistic terms, because it sets aside the autonomy (and human being) of the unborn child.

This argument can be elaborated through a demonstration that the Supreme Court's most recent abortion case, *Planned Parenthood v. Casey,* has evidenced an increasing lawlessness.

The "law" that theoretically empowers the justices to invalidate the acts of the political branches of government is the Constitution. In *Casey* the joint opinion specifically rejected the view that the justices, in interpreting the Constitution, are limited by the history and traditions of the American people. Instead, the justices believed themselves free to apply their "reasoned judgment" in interpreting the Constitution, even where such methodology leads them to reject the original understandings of the generations that framed, and lived under, the Constitution. The justices, in short, claim the unlimited and undefined authority to change the meanings of the document that is the basis of their authority.

Such a claim of authority itself can appear lawless, as "the Constitution" can become anything that a majority of Supreme Court justices believe it to be. America becomes a nation not of laws but of people. The joint opinion's response to this apparent fact of lawlessness was to grasp more power to assist the appearance, rather than the actuality, of lawfulness. Thus, the authors of the joint opinion claimed that they should not, based on a mere change of membership, overrule even an erroneous decision. Such overrulings, particularly where the membership changes were themselves a product of a political movement, would make it appear that the law was based merely on the membership of the court. Thus, the joint opinion affirmed the actuality of lawlessness — that the justices have the power and right to change the meaning of the Constitution — and then claimed the right to hide this actuality by maintaining an appearance of lawfulness.

A theory of judicial interpretation that permits the justices to cast aside original and long-standing historical understandings of the Constitution based on their own "reasoned judgment" undermines even the concept of an "erroneous" decision. The capacity of the Constitution to change with the "reasoned judgments" of the court's members suggests that all judgments are correct when made. "Error" is another word for an outdated rule, and is used when the current members of the court care enough about an issue to over-rule their predecessors. The "rule of law" becomes merely a prudential admonition to maintain the appearance of lawfulness.

The *Casey* joint opinion admits that the viability line has received "much criticism" and may seem "arbitrary," and that *Roe*'s balancing of the woman's right with fetal survival may be wrong. Nevertheless it reaffirms *Roe*'s fiat. Both *Roe* and *Casey* claimed to avoid deciding the moral status of abortion, or of the fetus, and thus claimed to avoid the moral or natural law questions raised by abortion. Thus, the central conflict between the woman's liberty and fetal life is never addressed in serious fashion in either *Roe* or *Casey*.

Under these circumstances, the court's claim of authority to use "reasoned judgment" in interpreting the Constitution appears to be an assertion of raw power to decide controversial public policy questions by invoking the "Constitution." The Constitution becomes a kind of seal of authority for whatever pronouncements the court wishes to make. It should be remembered that *Roe* was criticized not merely because it is "bad constitutional law," but rather "because it is not constitutional law and gives almost no sense of an obligation to try to be." *Casey* further undercut the court's sense of "obligation to trace its premises to the charter from which it derives its authority."

Thus, *Casey* stands as the most genuinely existentialist opinion of the Supreme Court. The joint opinion went beyond a rhetorical and doctrinal embrace of existentialism to the ultimate existentialist act of embracing the court's absolute power to recreate itself (and the Constitution) in each decision. Superficially, the court appeared to declare itself bound to precedent. On a deeper level, however, the court declared itself free from the shackles of text, history, and tradition, and bound by precedent only when, and if, it chose to be so bound. The only limitation the court acknowledged was the need to maintain its own power and reputation by providing society with a minimum degree of continuity and stability; within these broad bounds, the court could freely recreate both itself and the Constitution. The court solipstically declared itself as the primary referent of its decisions; the court's obligation to itself overrode any obligations to the historical Constitution, higher law, or the lawful acts of the political branches. The court justified such an orgy of self-absorbed power by declaring *itself* to be the virtual ground of being of the nation; the country's belief in itself would virtually collapse, suggested the joint opinion, if its faith in the court was somehow undermined. The court, we discover, is the savior of the nation.

Thus, *Casey* usurps the democratic process and seeks to lull people into the false view that life is not an "inalienable right" as stated in our Declaration of Independence. It is a malleable classification to be ultimately determined, if at all, by the Supreme Court, not by the people through our elected representatives based upon scientific facts.

This "lawless" usurpation must not go unchallenged. While any number of legal strategies may be proposed to eventually overturn *Roe* and its progeny, one way we can resist *Roe* and *Casey* right now is by establishing as a *scientific* fact the humanity of the human embryo and defending its right to life. Such a defense begins by understanding how the existence of a growing number of frozen and unchosen human embryos are being used as a justification by the National Institutes for Health to cynically ignore the existing federal funding ban on the destruction of human embryos, and to propose the funding of research on embryonic stem cells that can only be obtained by thawing and killing these embryos.[6]

6. Unless expressly instructed not to do so by Congress, it now appears that the National Institutes of Health (NIH), with President Clinton's support, intends to promulgate new federal regulations that will directly violate the existing federal law banning federal funding of destructive human embryonic stem cell research. See *NIH Guidelines for Research Involving Human Pluripotent Stem Cells,* 64 Fed. Reg. 67576 (December 2, 1999); Rick Weiss, "Embryonic Breathroughs? Stem Cell Studies Race Ahead as U.S. Policy Languishes," *Washington Post,* April 19, 2000, at A1.

In Section 510 of the FY 2000 Labor/HHS Appropriations Act [Pub. L. No. 106-13, Sec. 1000(a)(4)], the existing appropriations rider currently restricting the Department of Health and Human Services (DHHS) and its subordinates provides that *"none of the funds made available in this Act may be used for (1) the creation of a human embryo or embryos for research purposes; or (2) research in which a human embryo or embryos are destroyed, discarded, or knowingly subjected to risk of injury or death greater than that allowed for research on fetuses in utero under 45 C.F.R. [§] 46.208(a)(2) and section 498(b) of the Public Health Service Act (42 U.S.C. [§] 289g(b)]).*

On July 14, 1999, the President's Press Secretary, Mr. Lockhart, issued a statement wherein he stated: *NIH is putting in place guidelines and an oversight system that will ensure that the cells are obtained in an ethically sound manner. The President's 1994 ban on the use of federal funds for the creation of human embryos for research purposes will remain in effect. No other legal actions are necessary at this time, because it appears that human embryonic stem cells will be available from the private sector.* **Publicly funded research using these cells is permissible under the current Congressional ban on human embryo research.** (Emphasis added *in bold italics*)

Both NIH and the President are exclusively relying upon on a legal memorandum, dated January 15, 1999, issued by DHHS's Associate General Counsel Marcy Wilder, former Legal Director of the National Abortion Rights Action League and issued by DHHS's General Counsel, Harriett S. Rabb, claiming that despite the federal funding ban, federal funds can still pay for research using stem cells from deliberately destroyed human embryos so long as the federal funds do not pay for the act of destroying embryos. In a letter

Despite its high costs, practical uncertainties, low success rates, and physical difficulties, a growing number of infertile couples who cannot naturally conceive offspring now choose in vitro fertilization ("IVF").[7] With the

---

dated February 11, 1999, about 75 members of Congress requested Secretary Shalala to correct DHHS General Counsel's misinterpretation of the federal funding ban on destructive human embryo research. To date, the Secretary has ignored the request.

In September 1999, the National Bioethics Advisory Commission (NBAC) issued its advisory report to the President, entitled *Ethical Issues in Human Stem Cell Research*, recommending a lifting of the federal funding ban to permit federal agencies to fund research involving "the derivation and use of human embryonic stem cells from [human] embryos remaining after infertility treatments."

On January 31, 2000, Senators Specter of Pennsylvania and Harkin of Iowa introduced their proposed "Stem Cell Research Act of 2000" (S. 2015, the "Act") to effectively lift the federal funding ban in the case of research of "Human embryonic stem cells . . . derived only from embryos that otherwise would be discarded that have been donated from in vitro fertilization clinics with the written consent of the progenitors." On April 26, 2000, at the first hearing on the Act before the Senate Subcommittee on Labor, Health and Human Services, Education, and Related Agencies, Senator Brownback of Kansas, leading a growing coalition of Americans who oppose the killing of some human beings to provide medical research that may be helpful to other human beings, particularly when adult stem cell research promises to provide the same or greater benefits without the need to harm anyone, testified:

> In brief, the "Stem Cell Research Act of 2000" seeks to allow federal funding for researchers to kill living human embryos. Under this bill federal researchers would be allowed to obtain their own supply of living human embryos, which they would then be allowed to kill for research purposes. The very act of harvesting stem cells — or perhaps more accurately constructing so-called embryonic stem cells — from live human embryos results in the death of the embryo. Therefore, if enacted, this bill would result in the deliberate destruction of human embryos. This bill even violates current federal policy on fetal tissue, which allows harvesting of tissue only after an abortion was performed for other reasons and the unborn child is already dead. Under this bill, the federal government will use tax dollars to kill live embryos for the immediate and direct purpose of using their parts for research. Taxpayer funding of this research is problematic for a variety of reasons. First among those concerns is that, if Congress were to approve S. 2015, it would officially declare for the first time in our nation's history that government may exploit and destroy human life for its own or somebody else's purposes. This research is also problematic because it would use federal tax dollars to allow the government to procure, and therefore "own," a vast supply of living human embryos. The notion of "ownership," particularly by the federal government, of other human beings is deeply disturbing.

7. See John A. Robertson, "Embryos, Families, and Procreative Liberty: The Legal Structure of the New Reproduction," *S. Cal. L. Rev.* 59 (1968): 939, 942; Janette M. Puskar, "'Prenatal Adoption': The Vatican's Proposal to the In Vitro Fertilization Disposition Dilemma," *N.Y. L. Sch. J. Hum. Rts.* 14 (1998): 757. IVF costs are reported to range between

advancement of IVF technology, particularly the fact that fertility drugs given to women in IVF programs sometimes produce more embryos than can safely be implanted at any one time, it has become quite common to freeze the unused embryos for later thawing and implantation in a process known as cryopreservation.[8] Although this cryopreservation process may relieve the woman of the cost and physical burden of further egg retrievals in the IVF process while temporarily preserving the lives of the frozen embryos that would otherwise die for lack of implantation, it also brings along with it troubling medical, ethical, and legal issues, particularly when the parties divorce, die, or disagree about the disposition of the frozen embryos during the lengthy period between fertilization and implantation which cryopreservation permits.[9] I would now like to briefly review these issues and make a legislative proposal consistent with current constitutional law that resolves these issues in a manner most protective of human life.

$8,000 and $10,000 for a cycle of ovum retrieval and implantation, and up to $3,500 in medication costs per cycle. See Bette Harrison, "Special Delivery: A Baby," *Atlanta J.*, Dec. 21, 1997; Abigail Trafford, "Medicine's Money Back Warranty," *Wash. Post*, Aug. 5, 1997, at Health 6. The couple in the *Davis v. Davis* case spent $35,000 on IVF; the couple in *Kass v. Kass* spent over $75,000. David L. Theyssen, "Balancing Interests in Frozen Embryo Disputes: Is Adoption Really a Reasonable Alternative?" *Ind. L. J.* 74 (year?): 711, 734 n. 221. The IVF process can be stressful since the hormone injections can "produce pain, bloating and sharp mood swings" in the egg donor, in addition to the tedious blood tests and ultrasound examinations. *Time*, Nov. 14, 1994. Of the 400,000 couples who tried IVF, only 18 percent produced children. Denise Grady, "How to Coax New Life: Advances in Reproductive Techniques Give Couples Hope for Children Once Considered Impossible to Conceive," *Time*, Sept. 18, 1996. Even with considerable improvements in laboratory procedures, methods of egg retrieval, and techniques of ovarian stimulation, the highest reported success rates for pregnancy are between 25 and 36 percent, depending upon the age group involved. David Levan et al., "Pregnancy Potential of Human Oocytes — The Effect of Cryopreservation," *New Eng. J. Med.* 323 (1990): 1153. Live birth rates are lower still, at about 10 percent, due to miscarriages.

8. The process of in vitro fertilization involves a sophisticated treatment where mature eggs are obtained from the woman through a surgical procedure and fertilized outside the body. After fertilization occurs, they are placed back in the woman's uterus. Cryopreservation is the freezing of fertilized eggs in order to preserve them. See Clifton Perry and L. Kristen Schneider, "Cryopreserved Embryos: Who Shall Decide Their Fate?" *L. Legal Med.* 13 (1992): 463, 468.

9. See Knoppers and LeBris, "Recent Advances in Medically Assisted Conception: Legal, Ethical and Social Issues," *Am. J. L. & Med.* 4 (1991): 329. Without cryopreservation, all fertilized eggs must be implanted immediately or these human embryos will expire. See Marcia Joy Wurmbrand, "Frozen Embryos, Moral Social and Legal Implications," *S. Cal. L. Rev.* 59 (1986): 1079, 1083.

The Current Situation

There are more than ten million infertile couples in the United States.[10] In the last decade the infertility industry has grown from about thirty to over three hundred clinics earning revenues in excess of $1 billion. It is estimated that in the United States in 1999 more than 75,000 infants were born as a result of IVF — more than twice as many as will be available through traditional adoption. At the same time, more than 150,000 human embryos are now frozen, suspended in liquid nitrogen tanks (with more than 19,000 more frozen embryos estimated to be added to each year).[11] Yet while there are pages of adoption laws on the books in each state, only nine states — Louisiana, New Mexico, Florida, Pennsylvania, Kentucky, Kansas, Virginia, New Hampshire, and California — have enacted some legislation relating to IVF, and only three of these states — Louisiana, New Mexico, and Florida — regulate the disposition of the embryo in any way. Consequently, in most states the fate of most frozen embryos is left unpredictably open-ended.[12]

10. See Dominick Vetri, "Reproductive Technologies and United States Law," *Int'l. & Comp. L. Q.* 37 (1988): 505. Treatment for infertility varies from patient to patient. Depending upon the diagnosis, it may include timing of intercourse, hormone therapy to correct abnormalities in the natural menstrual cycle, intra-uterine insemination (IUI) to bypass problems with sperm or cervical mucous interactions, in vitro fertilization with embryo transfer, gamete or zygote intra-fallopian transfer (GIFT/ZIFT), frozen embryo transfer (FET), or intra-cytoplasmic sperm injection (ICSI). See IVF Phoenix Infertility Information Booklet, http://www.ihr.com/fertbook/treatment.htm.

11. Lori B. Andrews, "Embryonic Confusion," *Washington Post*, May 2, 1999, pp. B1, B4. "Not all embryos survive the freeze-thaw process. A 50% survival rate is considered reasonable. After the thaw, embryos retaining 50% or more of the cells they had before freezing are cultured and placed back in the uterus via a tube inserted in the cervix. The number returned varies with the desires of the patient under the guidelines of age categories; under 35 years old, up to four embryos, 35 years and older, up to six embryos. National statistics for women 39 or less is 27% per embryo transfer, for women over 39, 14% per embryo transfer. Delivery rates will be lower due to miscarriage." IVF Phoenix Infertility Information Booklet. Overall, "there is less than a 10% chance of creating a live birth from a frozen embryo." See Michelle F. Sublett, "Not Frozen Embryos: What Are They and How Should the Law Treat Them?" *Clev. St. L. Rev.* 38 (1990): 585, 593.

12. La. Rev. Stat. Ann. §9:123-33; N.M. Stat. Ann. §24-9A-1 to 7; Fla. Stat. Ann. §§742.11 et seq.; 18 Pa. Const. Stat. Ann. §3216(c)(1989); Ky. Rev. Stat. Ann. §311.715; Kan. Stat. Ann. §65-6702; N.H. Stats., Title XII, Chapter 168-B; VA St. §20-156 *et seq*. See generally Judith F. Daar, "Regulating Reproductive Technologies: Panacea or Paper Tiger," *Hous. L. Rev.* 34 (1997): 609.

The Louisiana law, passed in 1986, declares that an in vitro fertilized ovum is a "juridical person" that can be disposed of only through implantation. If IVF patients "fail to express their identity" or renounce parental rights, the physician is deemed to be the em-

The only federal law related to artificial reproductive technologies, like IVF, is the Fertility Clinic Success Rate and Certification Act of 1992.[13] It nei-

---

bryo's temporary guardian until adoptive implantations can occur. La. Rev. Stat. Ann. §9:123. In Louisiana, then, an agreement may not direct embryo dispositions other than implantation. Other options, such as a donation for research, or destruction, are prohibited. The federal constitutionality of this provision has not yet been tested.

The New Mexico statute prohibits all research involving embryos and fetuses, including IVF research. The statute allows the use of IVF to treat infertility as long as all the embryos are transferred to human recipients. N.M. Stat. Ann. §24-9A-1 to 7 (Michie 1997). Besides New Mexico, eight other states restrict embryo research indirectly, banning all research on "live" embryos or fetuses. Fla. Stat. Ann. §390.0111(6); Me. Rev. Stat. Ann. tit. 22. §1593 (West 1992); Mass. Ann. Laws ch. 112 §12j(a)(I) (Law Co-op. 1996); Mich. Comp. Laws Ann. §§333.2685, 333.2686, 333.2692 (West 1992); Minn. Stat. Ann. §145.222 subd. 1, 2 (West 1989); N.D. Cent. Code §§14-02.2-01, 14-02.2-02 (1991); 18 Pa. Cons. Stat. Ann. §3216(a) (Supp. 1995); R.I. Gen. Laws §11-54-1(a)-(c) (1994).

The Florida law is the only other law addressing prior embryo disposition agreements. Florida's law provides that couples undergoing IVF must enter into a written agreement that provides for the disposition of embryos in the event of death, divorce, or other "unforeseen circumstances"; and in the absence of a written agreement, the gamete providers are given joint dispositional authority. Fla. Stat. Ann. §742.17. The attempt in the first portion of this law to avert dispositional disputes by requiring prior agreements is effectively thwarted by the latter provision stating that in the absence of an agreement, the disagreeing gamete providers have joint authority — an invitation for judicial involvement without any legislative guidance.

The Pennsylvania statute requires all fertility clinics to file information concerning the location and staffing of each clinic, as well as the number of eggs fertilized, implanted, and destroyed. 18 Pa. Const. Stat. Ann. §3213(e). The Kentucky statute bars the use of public funds for the purpose of "obtaining an abortion" or the "intentional destruction of a human embryo." Ky. Rev. Stat. Ann. §311.715. The Kansas statute authorizes human embryo destruction by prohibiting any limitation on "the use of any drug or device that inhibits or prevents ovulation, fertilization or implantation of an embryo and disposition of the product of *in vitro* fertilization prior to implantation." Kan. Stat. Ann. §65-6702. The Virginia statute requires all fertility clinics to obtain a disclosure form executed by the patients indicating their knowledge of clinic practices, success rates, and other matters. Va. Code Ann. §54.1-2971.1 (Michie 1997). The New Hampshire statute restricts access to IVF and embryo transfers to women over twenty-one who meet stipulated medical criteria and requires a medical evaluation of all gamete providers. N.H. Rev. Stat. Ann. §168-B:13. The California laws make it "unlawful for anyone to knowingly use sperm, ova or embryos in assisted reproduction technology, for any purpose other than that indicated by the sperm, ova, or embryo provider's signature on a written consent form" (Cal. Penal Code §367g [West 1998]); and require the physician and surgeon who remove sperm or ova from a patient "to obtain the written consent of the patient," before the "sperm or ova are used for a purpose other than reimplantation in the same patient or implantation in the spouse of the patient" (Cal. Bus. & Prof. Code §2260 [West 1998]).

13. 42 U.S.C. §§201, 263a-1 to 263a-7 (Supp. 1996). The act requires the Centers for

ther governs nor regulates the disposition of frozen embryos. Nor are there any federal court cases establishing federal law on the subject of frozen embryos.

Other countries, such as Great Britain, have addressed this dilemma by instituting a law mandating the destruction of any frozen embryos that have been in a cryopreserved state for over five years.[14] In 1996, appalled by the imminent mass destruction of thousands of frozen embryos, the Vatican responded by suggesting "that married women volunteer to bring the embryos to term in 'prenatal adoption.'" At the time, there were approximately 9,300 fertilized embryos subject to destruction under the law. Of these 9,300 embryos, the clinics were able to reach the "parents" of 6,000 of the embryos, who exercised their rights under the law to extend the storage for another five years or donate the embryo for research or to another woman. The 3,300 remaining "potential infants" — in a chilling reminder of another Holocaust involving persons considered by their Nazi executioners to be "sub-human" — were thawed out, destroyed with saline solution, and incinerated with other biological waste.[15] Since that time, according to an April 14, 2000, report in the Reuters News Service, the Human Fertilization and Embryology

---

Disease Control to promulgate model certification procedures for fertility clinics and laboratories "to assure consistent performance of artificial reproductive technology procedures, quality assurance, and adequate record keeping at each certified embryo laboratory," as well as to standardize the reporting of pregnancy success rates. The reforms are minimal since the information required is otherwise available, neither laboratory certification nor clinic reporting are required by the Act, and the only "penalty" for failure to comply with the Act's recommendations is public identification as a program that has failed to do so. See Donna A. Katz, "My Egg, Your Sperm, Whose Preembryo? A Proposal for Deciding Which Party Receives Custody of Frozen Embryos," *Va. J. Soc. Pol'y & L.* 5 (1998): 623, 630.

14. Human Fertilisation and Embryology Act, 1990, ch. 37 §14 (Eng.). See generally Puskar, "'Prenatal Adoption,'" 757.

15. James Walsh, "A Bitter Embryo Imbroglio: Amid Dramatic Protests and Universal Unease, Britain Begins Destroying 3,300 Human Embryos," *Time*, Aug. 1996. The idea of "prenatal adoption" is neither new nor bizarre, as some IVF clinics require couples either to implant the frozen embryo in the natural mother, or donate it for implantation in another woman. For example, Louisiana and New Mexico law requires mandatory donation of the unused frozen embryo for purposes of implantation only, not destruction. While the constitutionality of a statute mandating "prenatal adoption" has not yet been determined, at least one commentator has concluded that such a statute would not infringe upon the federal privacy right because the "possibility of an anonymous hereditary tie" is at best only a psychological, not a physical burden and should therefore not be deemed an "undue burden" outweighing the state's interest in the potential life being protected by a mandatory pre-natal adoption statute. Puskar, "'Prenatal Adoption,'" pp. 62-63.

Authority, which regulates Great Britain's 120 fertility clinics, has said that it is difficult to know how many embryos have been destroyed because it is "a rolling program and the Authority is not notified when human embryos are thawed. But it estimates 51,000 embryos were thawed between April 1997 and March 1998. During the same period 152,504 embryos were created."

In Australia, the Infertility Treatment Act of 1984 has time restrictions similar to that of Britain, with the possibility of extension for reasonable grounds. The act requires that when implantation in the woman donor is not possible, the embryo should be made available to another woman with donor consent. The embryos can be destroyed if donors do not consent or withdraw their consent in writing. However, where the donors cannot be contacted, the government has the authority to order the hospital where the embryo is stored to implant the embryo in another woman.[16]

Germany avoids the problem entirely by prohibiting the freezing of embryos.[17]

Since 1978, when the first IVF baby, Louise Brown, was born in Great Britain, courts have also decided issues related to frozen human embryos in cases such as *Del Zios v. Columbia Presbyterian Medical Center*,[18] *York v.*

---

16. See Heidi Forster, "The Legal and Ethical Debate Surrounding the Storage and Destruction of Frozen Human Embryos: A Reaction to the Mass Disposal in Britain and the Lack of Law in the United States," *Wash. U. L. Q.* 76 (1998): 759, 761-64.

17. Ibid., p. 776, n. 28. While Germany prohibits the freezing of human embryos, it appears some researchers are seeking to avoid the violation by cryopreserving pronuclear oocytes in the prophase period prior to second meiosis and syngamy, which apparently can (upon being thawed) complete syngamy. See S. Hasani and E. Siebzehnubel, *Frozen Pronuclear Oocytes: Advantages for the Patients* (1999). Another way of avoiding the problem entirely would be the development of a reliable means of freezing and thawing unfertilized eggs, since a reliable means already exists for freezing and thawing sperm. Because the potential harm of freezing would occur before conception, and thus before the beginning of life, "right to life" concerns would not be implicated. However, the current technology for freezing and thawing unfertilized eggs is extremely unreliable. Furthermore, even after the technology develops to reliably freeze and thaw individual eggs, there will still be thousands of previously frozen embryos whose fate will have yet to be determined. Indeed, one commentator estimates that as many as 20,000 frozen embryos across the country may already be the subject of custody disputes. See Katz, "My Egg, Your Sperm, Whose Preembryo?" p. 674, n. 79. See also the article in *New Yorker* magazine, Aug. 9, 1999, "Annals of Reproduction: Eggs for Sale — Wanted: highly accomplished young women willing to undergo risky, painful medical procedure for very large sums."

18. *Del Zios* was the first unreported case involving frozen embryos. The Del Zioses filed suit when a supervising doctor at Columbia Presbyterian Medical Center intentionally destroyed the Del Zioses' human embryo obtained at the hospital through IVF because the doctor felt IVF constituted an unauthorized and "unwarranted practice which

Jones,[19] *Davis v. Davis, Kass v. Kass,* and *AZ v. BZ.*[20] In addition to these mostly appellate court decisions, there are at least two other trial court deci-

---

posed danger to any human life resulting from such experimentation." The jury rejected the Del Zioses' conversion claim for an unexplained reason, but returned a verdict for $50,000 for intentional infliction of emotional distress.

19. The dispute in *York* concerned one frozen fertilized embryo that the plaintiffs, Mr. and Mrs. York, sought to have released and transferred from an IVF clinic in Norfolk, Va., to another clinic in Los Angeles. 717 F. Supp. 421 (E. D. Va. 1989). The clinic refused to transfer the embryo and the Yorks sued for possession. The Yorks won when the court implicitly adopted the "embryo as property theory" (ibid. at 425) by noting that a bailor-bailee relationship was created (ibid.). The cryopreservation agreement between the Yorks and the clinic created a bailment because the clinic had legal possession of the embryo and had the duty to account for it (ibid. at 425). The court stated that when the purposes of the bailment relationship have terminated, "there is an absolute obligation to return the subject matter of the bailment to the bailor" (ibid.). The court found that the agreement between the parties recognized the Yorks' property rights and limited the clinic's rights as bailee (ibid. at 427). The court denied the clinic's motion to dismiss (ibid. at 429) and eventually the case settled. See generally Bill Davidoff, "Frozen Embryos: A Need for Thawing in the Legislative Process," *SMU L. Rev.* 47 (1993): 131.

20. *Davis* is the leading case that made its way up to the Tennessee Supreme Court, where the court decided the fate of seven frozen embryos. 842 S. W. 2d 588 (Tenn. 1992). A divorced couple, Mary Sue Davis and Junior Davis, were arguing over the disposition of their cryogenically preserved embryos resulting from IVF procedures. Mrs. Davis wanted to donate the remaining frozen embryos to another infertile couple, while Mr. Davis wanted them destroyed. The trial court, W. Dale Young presiding, based upon the expert testimony of the Nobel Prize–winning geneticist, Dr. Jerome LeJeune, held that the frozen embryos were "human beings" and awarded "custody" to Mrs. Davis so that she could have them implanted. At that time, Mrs. Davis wanted the frozen embryos to be implanted in her, and Mr. Davis wanted the embryos to remain frozen while he decided what to do (ibid. at 589). However, between 1989 when the case was decided by the trial court and 1992 when the Supreme Court of Tennessee rendered its decision, both parties had remarried and changed their positions.

The Court of Appeals reversed the trial court's finding that frozen embryos were human beings, likening them more to personal property and concluded that Mr. Davis had a "constitutionally protected right not to beget a child where no pregnancy has taken place" and that "there is no compelling state interest to justify ordering implantation against the will of either party" (ibid. at 598). The Court of Appeals remanded the case to the trial court for entry of an order giving both parties "joint control and equal voice over their disposition" because both parties shared an interest in their frozen embryos (ibid.).

The Supreme Court of Tennessee stated that although the Davises had an interest in the nature of ownership and disposition of the embryos, the interest was not a true property interest (ibid. at 597). The court concluded that frozen fertilized embryos deserve "special respect because of their potential for human life." The court also noted that the essential issue was whether the parties would become parents, not whether frozen embryos are "property" or "persons" (ibid. at 598). The court concluded that the answer to this dilemma "turns on

sions that suggest the need for state legislative action, if for no other reason than to avoid the increasing repetition of costly litigation, unpredictable re-

---

the parties' exercise of their constitutional right to privacy." The court discussed the cases where the Supreme Court held that the right to procreate was "one of the basic civil rights of man" (ibid. at 600, citing *Skinner v. Oklahoma*, 316 U.S. 535, 541[1942]). The court also noted that "the right of procreational autonomy is composed of two rights of limited but equal significance — the right to procreate and the right to avoid procreation" (ibid. at 601). The court held that in disputes concerning the disposition of a frozen embryo, a court should look first at "preferences of the progenitors" (ibid. at 601), and if there is a dispute, then a court should look at the prior agreement pertaining to the disposition of the embryo (ibid. at 592). If, in a case such as this one, there is no prior agreement, the court stated that it must resolve the dispute over "constitutional imports" (ibid. at 603) and weigh the interests of Mrs. Davis in her right to procreate and Mr. Davis in his right not to procreate (ibid. at 604). The court noted that "the party wishing to avoid procreation should prevail" if the other party has other reasonable means of procreating. If that party has no reasonable means of procreating, then the court will consider their argument for using the frozen embryo. In this case, Mrs. Davis wanted to donate her embryos to another couple, and the court held that in such a case, "the objecting party obviously has the greater interest and should prevail." Consequently, the Tennessee Supreme Court ruled that the Knoxville Fertility Clinic could destroy the Davises' human embryos.

The dispute in *Kass* involved the issue of the disposition of five frozen fertilized embryos (663 N.Y. S. 2d 581 [App. Div. 1997]). The parties in this case — now divorced — were arguing over the disposition of the five frozen embryos (FN153). However, unlike the situation in the *Davis* case, when the Kasses underwent IVF treatments, they signed an informed consent document which provided in pertinent part: "In the event that we no longer wish to initiate a pregnancy or are unable to make a decision regarding the disposition of our stored, frozen pre-zygotes, we now indicate our desire for the disposition of our pre-zygotes and direct the IVF Program to: . . . (b) Our frozen pre-zygotes may be examined by the IVF Program for biological studies and be disposed of by the IVF Program for approved research investigation as determined by the IVF Program" (ibid. at 584).

During the divorce proceedings, the parties executed a document that set forth their understanding of what was previously agreed to in the informed consent document as to the disposition of the remaining frozen embryos (ibid. at 584). However, Mrs. Kass had a change of heart and wanted to have the embryos implanted in *her* uterus (ibid. at 584-85). Mr. Kass wanted to have them turned over for embryo research, as provided for in the informed consent document.

The trial court awarded Mrs. Kass the five embryos for implantation (ibid. at 585). The trial court first reasoned that embryos enjoy the status of something between human life and property. The court stated that, just as in in vivo fertilization, a father's right ends at the moment of fertilization. The court concluded that the issue of embryo disposition is a matter exclusively within the mother's discretion. The court further found that the informed consent document agreed to by the parties was not dispositive and agreed that, in the event of a divorce, a court would determine the issue of disposition. Therefore, the trial court held that Mrs. Kass was to determine the fate of the five frozen embryos.

The Appellate Division reversed and held that the informed consent document and

sults, unacceptable delays, public intrusion in private lives, and ongoing familial disruption.[21] At present, relying on various rationales for their deci-

---

the uncontested divorce instrument clearly stated the parties' intent that in the event of a divorce, any remaining embryos were to be donated for scientific research (ibid. at 590). The court first criticized the lower court's analysis and stated that it had committed a "fundamental error" (ibid. at 585). The court stated that the Supreme Court was wrong to "[equate] a prospective mother's decision whether to undergo implantation of pre-zygotes which are the product of her participation in an IVF procedure with a pregnant woman's right to exercise exclusive control over the fate of her non-viable fetus."

Rather, the court found that the first inquiry should be whether the parties had made an "expression of mutual intent which governs the disposition of the pre-zygotes under the circumstances in which the parties find themselves" (ibid. at 585). The court relied on the *Davis* decision where the Supreme Court of Tennessee stated that a critical factor in determining the disposition of frozen embryos is whether there was a prior written agreement (ibid. at 587). The *Kass* court found that because the Kasses executed the informed consent document, which was clear and unambiguous, the embryos would have to be disposed of as provided for in that agreement (ibid. at 588). The court also noted that Mrs. Kass did not meet the evidentiary standards to permit the balancing test, as used in *Davis v. Davis*, which balances the parties' interests in using the embryos (ibid. at 590). The court concluded that "the decision to attempt to have children through IVF procedures and the determination of the fate of cryopreserved pre-zygotes resulting therefrom are intensely personal and essentially private matters which are appropriately resolved by the prospective parents rather than the courts." The court determined that if the parties had entered into a prior agreement indicating their mutual intent regarding the disposition of any unused frozen embryos, then a court must not interfere. Therefore, because the Kasses had executed the informed consent document indicating that in the event of any unforeseen circumstances, the court held that the Kass embryos be retained by the IVF Program for scientific research.

On May 7, 1998, the Appellate Division's decision was affirmed on appeal to the New York Court of Appeals, where the court held that the parties' agreement providing for donation to the IVF Program controls the issue. 696 N.E. 2d 174 (N.Y. 1998).

In *AZ v. BZ*, the most recent appellate decision involving frozen human embryos, the trial court entered a permanent injunction in favor of the husband, prohibiting the wife "from utilizing" frozen "preembryos" held in cryopreservation at an in vitro fertilization (IVF) clinic. Wife appealed. Transferring the case on its own motion, the Supreme Judicial Court of Massachusetts, addressing an issue of first impression [in Massachusetts], held that a consent form signed by the parties on the one hand and the clinic on the other, providing that, on the parties' separation, the frozen human "preembryos" were to be given to the wife for implantation, was unenforceable. While saying nothing about the humanity of the human embryos involved, the Court simply affirmed the permanent injunction below stating: "In this case, we are asked to decide whether the law of the Commnwealth may compel an individual to become a parent over his or her contemporaneous objection. The husband signed this consent form in 1991. Enforcing the form against him would require him to become a parent over his present objection to such an undertaking. We decline to do so." 431 Mass. 150, 162, 725 Ne.E.2d 1051, 1059. Conse-

sions, the general trend has been for the courts to side with the party seeking the destruction of the human embryos either on contractual grounds or on the ground that the interest in avoiding procreation trumps all other asserted interests, including the state's interest in protecting human life and the parties' contractual rights.[22]

---

quently, the human embryos in this case remain frozen absent an agreement by the parties as to what to do with them. The *AZ* Court provided no further guidance except to say: *We express no view regarding whether an unambiguous agreement between two donors concerning the dispostion of frozen preembryos could be enforced over the contemporaneous objection of one of the donors, when such an agreement contemplated destruction or donation of the preembryos either for research or implantation in a surrogate. We also recognize that agreements among donors and IVF clinics are essential to clinic operations. There is no impediment to the enforcement of such contracts by the clinics or by the donors against the clinics, consistent with the principles of this opinion.*

21. The unreported trial court frozen embryo cases are the New Jersey case of *J.B. v. M.B.* and the Michigan case of *Bohn v. Ann Arbor Reproductive Medicine Associates.*

In the New Jersey case of *J.B. v. M.B.*, there was no written agreement and it was the Catholic husband who sought to bar his former wife from destroying the frozen embryos they produced while they were still married. The court rejected his claim to assume all parental responsibilities in order to preserve the embryos to implant in another woman or donate them to an infertile couple because "he is quite healthy and fully able to father a child . . . in such a case[, like *Davis*,] where the party seeking control of the frozen embryos intends merely to donate them to another couple, the objecting party has the greater interest and should prevail."

The *Bohn* case in Michigan involved a suit against a fertility clinic by a former wife for custody of three frozen embryos conceived by IVF while she was married to her former husband so that she could have the embryos implanted in her as provided in her alleged written contract with the fertility clinic, which was signed only by her, not her former husband. The divorced husband intervened in the case arguing that the implantation of the embryos in his former wife violates his "[constitutional] right not to procreate" and that there was no agreement between himself and his former wife giving her exclusive custody over the remaining embryos to do with them as she in her sole discretion may decide. The wife seeks to protect the lives of the embryos while protecting her right to affirmatively procreate, which under the facts of this case she argues can most likely be accomplished through the implantation of the remaining three embryos in her uterus. The trial court held that "neither [the former wife or the former husband] have a unilateral contractual right to take possession of the embryos, and until such time as they agree on a disposition, the embryos may remain [in their cryopreserved state]. The trial court further held that the Michigan Child Custody Act, by its terms and intent, does not apply to frozen embryos. Finally, the *Bohn* court held that the objecting gamete provider "has a constitutional right not to beget offspring, and, therefore, has the right to veto any use of the embryos to produce more children" (ibid. at 12). In an unpublished decision issued in December 1999, the Michigan Court of Appeals affirmed the decision and urged the Michigan Legislature to provide statutory guidance to the courts as to how to proceed in cases involving frozen human embryos.

22. The American Bar Association, at its 1998 Meeting in Nashville, Tenn., consid-

The cases essentially turn on two questions. The first is, what is the legal status of the frozen embryo? The second is, ought this status be determined: by the gamete providers as a matter of private contractual law or by the state as a matter of public policy, particularly when the gamete providers either disagree, die, divorce, or are otherwise unavailable? Regarding the status of the frozen embryo, there are four basic theories: (1) the "Human Life" theory that the frozen embryo is a human being deserving the equal protection of the laws against homicide; (2) the "Pure Property" theory that the frozen embryo is merely property to be dealt with under common law contract and personal property principles; (3) the "Special Status" theory that the frozen embryo deserves "special respect" as against the claims of the non-gamete providers, but not possessing rights sufficient to limit the procreative or contractual rights of the gamete providers themselves; and (4) the "Constitutional Rights" theory, based upon analogies to distinguishable Supreme Court "right to privacy" decisions protecting abortion and contraception, that the unborn have no constitutionally protectible right to life, but a gamete provider does have a right "not to procreate" that trumps any constitutional, statutory or contractual rights against the destruction of a human embryo prior to implantation that the state or any other gamete provider may assert. Each theory has its proponent and critics.[23]

---

ered adopting a policy statement, proposed by the Family Law Section (Report No. 106), about frozen embryo disposition. The ABA indefinitely postponed the policy. The proposed ABA policy states that it is intended for use "in cases of marriage dissolution where the couple has previously stored frozen embryos with the intent to procreate." The policy suggests that if the marriage has dissolved, the couple is in disagreement about the fate of the embryos, and there is no pre-procedural agreement, "the party wishing to proceed in good faith and in a reasonable time, with gestation to term, and to assume parental rights and responsibilities should have possession and control of all the frozen embryos."

23. There are more than 320 law review articles on the legal controversies surrounding frozen human embryos. See generally, Puskar, " 'Prenatal Adoption,' " pp. 765-66; Katz, "My Egg, Your Sperm, Whose Preembryo?" pp. 634-39 ["The [Constitutional] theory . . . is distinct from, but in accordance with the [Special Status theory]. . . . Because the Supreme Court [denied *certiorari* in *Davis v. Davis*, 842 S.W. 2d 588 (Tenn. 1992), *cert., denied* 507 U.S. 911 (1993) and] has not decided a case involving the custody of [human embryos], the statement of its view regarding their status is based upon the extrapolation from the Court's analysis of the status of the unborn." In *Roe v. Wade*, 410 U.S. 113 (1973), the Court held that the word "person" "has application only post-natally . . . [and,] as used in the Fourteenth Amendment, does not include the unborn" (ibid. at 157-58). Logically then, if the word "person" does not apply to the fetus, which is at a considerably more advanced stage of development, it does not apply to a human embryo that is not even located in the uterus.]

On the other hand, the Constitutional theory is limited in its application to human

Those who hold that the embryo is a living human being seek protective legislation, like the laws of Louisiana and New Mexico, permitting "prenatal adoption" of frozen embryos and prohibiting the intentional destruction of human embryos.[24] Such proponents also support judicial application of the "best interests of the child" standard for determining which of the gamete providers ought to have custody of the frozen embryos, regardless of any written agreements the gamete providers may have to destroy or donate the embryos for destructive research. Based upon Dr. Jerome LeJeune's expert genetics testimony calling the human embryo "early human beings" and "tiny persons," and equating the destruction of a frozen embryo with death from a "concentration can," the trial court in the *Davis v. Davis* case adopted the Human Life theory and gave custody to the mother who wished to preserve the lives of her frozen embryos over her husband's desire to destroy them because they had subsequently been divorced.

Those who hold that frozen embryos are "pure property" generally support legislation that (a) affirms the gamete providers' joint decisional authority over their frozen embryos, with or without a pre-conception agreement; (b) requires them to enter an agreement providing for the broad range of dispositional alternatives, including destruction, storage, donation for research, and donation to another infertile couple; and (c) ensures the enforce-

---

embryos ex utero because *Roe* has been held to be limited to abortion, and, "outside the context of abortion, the states can protect the unborn human being at every stage of development." See generally, Clarke D. Forsythe, "Human Cloning and the Constitution," *Valparaiso U. L. Rev.* 32 (1998): 469, 500-502, n. 141, and accompanying text ["Recently, Indiana became the twenty-sixth state to treat as a homicide the killing of an unborn human being at some stage of gestation when it enacted a law, over the Governor's veto, to treat the killing of an unborn child as homicide whether the child was born alive or not. In addition, Michigan and Wisconsin enacted legislation in 1998 to protect the unborn child ("embryo" and "fetus") at all stages of gestation. Thus, states continue to extend legal protection to the unborn human being throughout gestation, and, outside the context of abortion, a remarkable legal and legislative consensus exists across at least thirty-eight states that the life of a human being begins at fertilization or conception."]

24. For Louisiana, see La. Rev. Stat. Tit. 9 §§121-133, Tit. 14 §87.2, Tit. 40 §1299.35.13, 1299.35.18; for New Mexico, see N.M. Stat. Ann. §24-9A-1 to 7; for several other states that recognize the human embryo as a legal "person" or specifically forbid the killing or experimenting upon the human embryo, see Me. Rev. Stat. Tit. 22 §§1593-1595 (Maine); Mass. Gen. Laws, ch. 112 §12J (a) et seq. (Massachusetts); Mich. Comp. Laws §§333.2685-333.2691 (Michigan); Minn. Stat. §§145.421-145.422 (Minnesota); N.H. Rev. Stat. Tit. 12 §§168-B:13–168-B:15 (New Hampshire); N.D. Cent. Code §§14-02.2-01–14-02.2-02(5) (North Dakota); Pa. Cons. Stat. Tit. 18 §§3216(a)-3216(c) (Pennsylvania); R.I. Gen. Laws §§11-54-1(a)-11-54-1(f) (Rhode Island); Utah Code Ann. §76-7-310, 76-7-314 (Utah).

ability of such prior directives. In the absence of prior agreement, such "pure property" proponents generally assert that courts should prohibit use of frozen embryos by either party without the consent of the other. Such a Pure Property theory was the approach taken in *Davis v. Davis* by the Tennessee Court of Appeals in reversing the trial court decision based upon the Human Life theory.

Those who hold the Special Status theory take an intermediate view between the Pure Property theory and the Human Life theory. The frozen embryo is not given the full status afforded a human being, but is not considered pure property either. According to this theory, the embryo is given greater respect than human tissue because of its potential life. Proponents of this theory respect the embryo as a "symbol of human life." The American Fertility Society has adopted this position. The Special Status theory was the approach adopted by the Tennessee Supreme Court in affirming the result, if not the reasoning, of the Tennessee Court of Appeals in *Davis v. Davis*.

A Life-Protective Proposal of Law re Frozen Human Embryos

Based upon the unpredictable, inconsistent, and unduly costly results described above, the courts and commentators appear to uniformly agree that the United States, on the federal and state levels, should adopt a legislative framework regulating the cryogenic preservation and implantation of human embryos. Unfortunately, many of the proposals ignore the humanity of the human embryo by recommending that human embryos be likened to property, not people, with no protectible legal interests of their own.[25]

In opposition to those proposals, the following elements of a more life-protective proposal of law regulating the cryogenic preservation of human embryos on a current and prospective basis are proposed:

1. As already established in thirty-eight states, the life of the human being would be expressly acknowledged as a scientific fact to begin at fertilization or conception, not at implantation.[26]

25. See Kimberly E. Diamond, "Cryogenics, Frozen Embryos and the Need for New Means of Regulation: Why the U.S. Is Frozen in Its Current Approach," *N.Y. Int'l. L. Rev.* 11 (1998): 77.

26. See Paul B. Linton, "Planned Parenthood v. Casey: The Flight from Reason in the Supreme Court," *St. Louis U. Pub. L. Rev.* 13 (year?): 15, 120, App. B (collecting legislation and caselaw from 38 states); Forsythe, "Human Cloning and the Constitution," p. 469, 501 n. 148.

2. As already established in Louisiana, the ex utero human embryo would be deemed a "juridical person" entitled to pursue its continued development until its term in the organism of its biological or adoptive mother. If IVF patients "fail to express their identity" or renounce parental rights, the physician is deemed to be the embryo's temporary guardian until an adoptive implantation can occur.

3. As already established in New Mexico, human embryos can only be disposed of through implantation, not intentional destruction or through destructive human embryo research.

4. Prospectively, the cryopreservation of a human embryo shall only be permitted as needed to preserve its life until implantation can occur.

5. The pursuit of its continued development until its term in the organism of its biological or adopted mother must be offered to each human embryo before another embryo may be conceived.

6. As already established in Australia, existing cryopreserved human embryos may only be thawed and allowed to deteriorate after five years, if and only if the gamete providers do not earlier consent to an extension of this time or to their implantation in the organism of the biological or adopted mother, and no one can be found by the custodian of the human embryo willing to accept implantation of the human embryo and assume parental responsibility for it.

7. Agreements for the destruction of a human embryo, or the donation of a human embryo for biological or medical research not designed to evaluate, protect, or restore the health of that human embryo shall be unenforceable as violative of public policy, and not entitled to government funding of any kind.

8. No human embryo can be intentionally created for or submitted to any exploitation whatsoever, including being created for any investigational research purpose not intended to diagnose or improve the life or health of the embryo or individual biological parent, and which results in the destruction of the embryo.[27]

9. Prior to any IVF procedure, all IVF providers must obtain the gamete providers' signatures on a written disclosure form and dispositional agreement that fully informs the gamete providers of the law requiring the implantation of all human embryos so conceived, as well as the

27. See Christine L. Feiler, "Human Embryo Experimentation: Regulation and Relative Rights," *Fordham L. Rev.* 69 (1998): 2435, proposing a federal statute to prohibit the creation and exploitation of research embryos and correct the problems identified in existing legislation.

costs, risks, and probabilities for success involved in IVF procedures being used, and the time for deterioration of cryopreserved embryos should such preservation be necessary to maintain the viability of the cryopreserved embryos prior to implantation.

The foregoing proposal offers a moral and juridical framework for decisions, decrees, and ordinances regulating the ex utero creation and use of human embryos using artificial reproductive technologies. It is inspired by the expert testimony of Dr. Jerome Lejeune, as presented before the trial court in *Davis v. Davis*, that the human embryo is a human being.[28] In the true words of the trial court's opinion in *Davis v. Davis*, based on that compelling testimony:

> [C]ryogenically preserved embryos are human beings. . . . human embryos are not property. Human life begins at conception. Mr. and Mrs. Davis have produced human beings, *in vitro*, to be known as their child or children. For domestic relations purposes, no public policy prevents the continuing development of the common law as it applies to . . . human beings existing as embryos, in vitro, in this domestic relation case. The common law doctrine of parens patriae ["the power of the sovereign to watch over the interests of those incapable of protecting themselves"] controls children, in vitro. It is to the manifest best interests of the child or children, in vitro, that they be available for implantation. It serves the best interests of the child or children, in vitro, for their mother . . . to be permitted the opportunity to bring them to term through implantation.[29]

An Invitation to Join DO NO HARM: The Coalition of Americans for Research Ethics

On Thursday, July 1, 1999, the Center for Bioethics and Human Dignity publicly released its statement in opposition to human embryonic stem cell re-

28. See Dr. Jerome Lejeune, *The Concentration Can: When Does Human Life Begin? An Eminent Geneticist Testifies* (San Francisco: Ignatius Press, 1992). Part 5 of this work contains a "Proposal of Law on the Health of the Human Person," similar to the one proposed above, which was presented to the French Parliament on May 20, 1990, with the support of Dr. LeJeune.

29. For a more complete understanding of the trial court's decision in *Davis v. Davis*, please write for a copy of the Christian Legal Society's helpful booklet, "The Custody Dispute over Seven Human Embryos: The Testimony of Professor Jerome Lejeune, M.D., Ph.D."

search during a press conference in Washington, D.C. The Center has been collaborating with Senator Sam Brownback and numerous other individuals and organizations in an initiative directed against federally funded medical research involving the destruction of human embryos. Senator Brownback stated that he is committed to ensuring that the current ban against government funding of such research be interpreted and upheld as proscribing research on human embryonic stem cells.

The statement, entitled *On Human Embryos and Stem Cell Research: An Appeal for Legally and Ethically Responsible Science and Public Policy,* has already been signed by a broad coalition of more than a hundred health-care leaders, bioethicists, legal experts, including Dr. Koop, Dr. Stevens, Dr. Frank Young, Dr. Edmund Pellegrino, Dr. Hook, Dr. Kilner, Dr. Cameron, Dr. Rae, Dr. Mitchell, and many others.[30]

Based upon the principles set forth in the statement, "Do No Harm," The Coalition of Americans for Research Ethics (CARE) has now been formed with the mission to become a

> growing national coalition of patients, researchers, health-care professionals, bio-ethicists, legal professionals, and others dedicated to the promotion of scientific research and health care which does no harm to human life while advancing legally and ethically responsible science, health care and public policy.

The initial three objectives of the DO NO HARM Coalition are:

1. To advance the development of medical treatments and therapies that do not require the destruction of human life, including the human embryo.
2. To educate and inform public policy makers and the general public regarding these ethically acceptable and medically promising areas of research and treatment.
3. To support continuation of the federal law prohibiting the federal fund-

---

30. The statement acknowledges that stem cell research promises great good and is a worthy scientific priority as long as it is pursued using ethical means. Obtaining stem cells from people without seriously harming people in the process can be ethical. However, obtaining stem cells from human embryos cannot be ethical because it necessarily involves destroying those embryos. The statement argues that funding embryonic stem cell research would violate existing law and policy, be unethical, and is scientifically unnecessary. A copy of the statement, its executive summary, and a list of its signatories may be found at DO NO HARM's website, http://www.stemcellresearch.org.

ing of research that would require the destruction of human life, including the human embryo.

This effort is required because support for human embryo research has been steadily growing since 1995, when the federal funding ban on destructive human embryonic research was first imposed. The National Bioethics Advisory Commission has issued its report to the President endorsing federal funding for destructive human embryonic stem cell research provided that the existing ban on such funding be first lifted by Congress. The National Institutes for Health has indicated that it intends to ignore the federal funding ban and in December 1999 published its proposed regulatory guidelines for selecting the human embryos that may be destroyed to obtain the embryonic stem cell for research use. The recently created Coalition for Urgent Research (CURE), a lobbying coalition representing victims of twenty-eight diseases, is campaigning to overturn the research ban, saying fairness and compassion for disease victims that may be helped by research using the stem cells of destroyed human embryos should prevail.

As recently stated in *Christianity Today* (Editorials, July 12, 1999), "the coming battle over research on human embryos promises to be a defining moment in bioethics and is a struggle that should engage those who truly value all human life." As it does, those who believe in the inalienable right to life for all human beings, including such beings in their embryonic stage of human life, should be inspired by the words of the Dutch Christian reformer, Abraham Kuyper, who said:

> When principles that run against your deepest convictions begin to win the day then battle is your calling, and peace has become sin; you must at the price of deepest peace, lay your convictions before friend and enemy with all the fire of your faith.

PART IV

HEALTH CARE

Medicine and the Challenge of Change

David L. Stevens, M.D.

After two nights on call and a full day in the office, Janet hurriedly sorted through the mail. Her colleague, Frank, was taking a few days off before Janet would take her turn attending the state medical association meeting. She was looking forward to seeing old friends, and especially to getting four consecutive good nights of sleep!

Janet grabbed the meeting packet from her desk where it had lain for two weeks. As she glanced over the agenda items, she was shocked. The first proposal on the agenda, submitted by Bill Engstrom, was that the association adopt a *neutral* stance on physician-assisted suicide.

Janet had gone to medical school with Bill twenty years ago. For the last few years, she had noticed his name in the news as one of the state's leading proponents of physician-assisted suicide. All the same, she couldn't believe that Bill had actually sponsored the motion on the ballot. A neutral position by the association would add enormous impetus to legalizing physician-assisted suicide in the state. What could she ever do on such short notice?

*   *   *

"Wow! What a great rotation!" John thought to himself, "Well, that settles the big question. I'm going to specialize in OB-GYN." During his time in obstetrics-gynecology, John had discovered that he loved delivering babies — even in the middle of the night. He bubbled over as he shared his thoughts with Melinda, one of the women in his Christian Medical & Dental Society campus group. But Melinda's first comment threw ice water on his enthusiasm.

"I hear it is almost impossible to get an OB-GYN residency unless you are willing to do abortions," she said. "One of my pro-life friends, who ranked in the top ten percent of her class, listed ten residencies and didn't get a single match. She was way out on a limb trying to find a residency with all the good slots gone!"

*   *   *

Karen was so upset that she couldn't sleep. She thought she knew Dr. Little pretty well after taking care of his admissions in the ICU for over ten years. That's why Karen couldn't believe Dr. Little ordered ten milligrams of morphine and directed that the ventilator be removed from Mrs. Kushe. Mrs. Kushe was seventy-two years old. She had suffered a stroke five days ago, had been aspirated, and now required ventilator support. She was paralyzed on her left side and had been semi-comatose.

But Karen had seen some improvement in the last twenty-four hours. Mrs. Kushe now responded to verbal stimuli, and followed with her eyes as Karen moved around the room. Karen told Dr. Little that Mrs. Kushe would die if she were given the morphine and had the ventilator removed. "I realize what will happen," he replied curtly. He confided that Mrs. Kushe's daughter, a busy lawyer, had assured him that her mother would not want to live paralyzed. The daughter had requested that all "heroic" efforts be stopped.

"I don't have any choice," Dr. Little offered. "The daughter has power of attorney for health care."

Karen refused to be part of killing a partially paralyzed patient who still had a reasonable chance to live. So Dr. Little gave the night shift nurse the assignment. Mrs. Kushe was probably dying right now.

Karen tortured herself with second thoughts. "Should I have done more? Should I have taken the issue to the administration or the hospital medical director? Did I just stand by and allow this woman's life to be taken from her? Was Dr. Little ethically justified or dead wrong? Have I put my job in jeopardy by refusing to carry out his orders?"

*   *   *

If only the above scenarios were made up. Unfortunately, they are composites of frequent phone calls and conversations that the Christian Medical & Dental Society (CMDS) has with physicians, nurses, physician assistants, students, and patients' families. These and hundreds of similar stories show that ethics is no longer an abstract set of issues for health-care professionals.

Increasingly, health-care professionals face agonizing quandaries on a shifting ethical landscape. It is hard enough to keep abreast of rapidly developing technology, much less determine the ethics of its applications. Issues once thought settled are now *unsettling*. Euthanasia, abortion, homosexuality, and even pedophilia are being redefined as noble "choices."

Health-care providers are overwhelmed by managed care's hurricane force of change. Seemingly overnight, medicine underwent a transformation from a calling to a *business*. Many doctors have lost their autonomy. Business interests pressure nurses to do more with less help as paperwork piles up. This war zone of business and bureaucracy has made casualties of patient care and professional satisfaction. Christians are encouraged to practice New Age medicine such as therapeutic touch. Others, such as obstetrical nurses expected to aid abortions to gain promotions, work under daily pressure to compromise their morality. Nurses find themselves increasingly caught in the middle between doctor, patient, and family. Today health professionals face similar and unique challenges, packing the workplace with mounting stress.

Uniquely Equipped

In the midst of the tumult, many health-care professionals take a defensive posture. They attempt to survive by avoiding conflict. But God has placed Christians into health care for *such a time as this*. Like Daniel and Esther, Christian physicians and nurses can use their positions to influence and alter the natural course of events. The need has never been greater nor the issues more vital. In this pivotal moment, God has uniquely equipped health-care professionals with several weapons for the ethical wars.

Knowledge

The first weapon is the armor of *knowledge*. Health-care professionals hold the knowledge of science and technology that is interwoven into almost every controversy. They can answer questions such as: "Is a mother's health really a justification for a partial-birth abortion?" "Is there a better alternative to killing embryos to obtain stem cells?" "Is severe pain controllable with modern methods of analgesia, sedatives, and anesthesia?" "Does the fetus feel pain during a second trimester abortion?" When knowledge is ammunition, the answers to these questions have a powerful effect on the battle.

Health-care professionals hold *secret* knowledge. No one else has similar access to the hushed halls of hospitals, clinics, and nursing homes. No one else stands at the bedside or beside the exam table as a patient grapples with an unplanned pregnancy or receives a diagnosis of terminal illness. No one else has agonized about whether to put a patient on a ventilator. No one else has titrated the morphine to decrease the air hunger when a patient is taken off a ventilator to die. Health-care providers have sympathetically shared experiences with their chronically and terminally ill patients are on. Patients value and desire this secret knowledge of what lies ahead.

Experience

Health-care professionals have the proven weapon of *experience.* They have fought to apply ethical principles to clinical situations and have accumulated the gripping stories that can sway the hearts of decision-makers.

Physician-assisted suicide advocates state that a competent patient who is terminally ill with less than six months to live and in uncontrollable suffering should have the right to die with a physician's help. This claim has several presuppositions: It assumes that doctors can accurately predict that a patient has only six months to live. A health-care professional can draw on *knowledge,* citing a recent survey revealing that half of Oregon's doctors admit that they cannot accurately predict that a patient has only six months to live. An experienced clinicians knows that patients often live much longer than anticipated, and that new treatments can unexpectedly prolong their lives. Relating a personal *experience* is more convincing to an individual than reams of data.[1] Through a story, the listener emotionally identifies with the situation as a husband, wife, or critically ill child. Voting levers, poll questionnaires, and personal decisions are often pulled by heartstrings. *Data changes knowledge, but stories change hearts.*

---

1. I could tell the powerful story of my mother-in-law. She had metastatic breast cancer, suffered a light stroke, and had severe obstructive respiratory disease. The cancer was in her bones, she was not eating, her lips were blue from her lung problem, and her weight was down to 85 pounds. Her primary doctor and specialists advised us that we should come home from Kenya to see her one last Christmas before she died. As a physician, knowing her condition, I agreed that she was unlikely to survive six months. I believed it to the extent that I spent $3,000 of our meager savings for my wife and me to travel to the United States. We had a great Christmas. My mother-in-law ultimately died. But it was fifteen wonderful years later!

Influence

Through the relationships that health-care professionals form, they gain the weapon of *influence*. Caregivers have a unique relationship with patients and families. They listen to and examine each patient. They order and perform tests, plan and administer therapy, and control information. Patients and families look to these experts for advice and are profoundly influenced by it. These relationships can yield confidence, anger, hope, despair, laughter, tears, or a mass of conflicting emotions. A patient and family's entire day in the hospital centers around the moments they have with each doctor, nurse, or caregiver. This influential relationship is built upon and sustained by *trust*, a powerful weapon in ethical wars.

Health-care professionals also hold influence within the unique fraternity of health-care providers. Intense training, special knowledge, experience, and high stress create a bond among caregivers. This unity is built on an unspoken belief that outsiders cannot fully understand this world and have little right to influence it. So, caregivers look to colleagues as they consider their positions on ethical issues.[2]

Respect

The fourth major weapon is *respect*. Health-care professionals enjoy a high level of respect from patients and the public, especially caregivers perceived as

2. Health-care professionals also have singular influence because of their relationships with third-party players, such as managed-care organizations, insurance companies, and the government. Unfortunately, this influence has markedly decreased in the last decade, as these entities have capitalized on the fact that money leverages power. They have cornered the market by offering cheaper health-care costs to businesses and legislators, and then dictating terms to providers.

Cowed by the industry players' threat of "accept our terms or lose your patient base," doctors are working much harder for a lot less. Health-care inflation has dropped, but only at the expense of "dumbing down" the profession and converting it to a business model of efficiency and production quotas. This has resulted in less-trained caregivers, fewer providers, and scores of personnel at the peak of their knowledge and efficiency leaving their professions out of frustration and anger.

The pendulum may be beginning to swing back in some areas, as health-care providers are speaking out and banding together to protect their interests. Their influence with the industry players is growing once again, but sometimes at the expense of their professional integrity. Though less potent, this influence with players still can be used in ethical battles.

genuinely caring, sacrificial, and competent. This is where Christian care-givers have the edge. With patients, colleagues, and media contacts, they should emphasize their volunteer work for the poor in domestic and international missions, or similar endeavors. This is not to forsake humility, but to build credibility, which is key to the influence and respect that opens doors to the Christian message.

Direct Impact

Health-care givers also must be involved in the ethical war because the outcomes of that war will directly impact them. They will be asked to apply the "new ethics" to their own patients and practice. This is already happening, as doctors are being asked to turn off ventilators.

One such case was this: Georgette Smith was accidentally shot by her mother, who was aiming at Georgette's boyfriend. The man had suggested that the ailing mother be put in a nursing home against her will. The neck wound made Georgette a quadriplegic dependent on a ventilator.[3] After a psychiatrist declared her competent, Georgette petitioned the court to have the ventilator removed. The court said she had the right to refuse care but made no comment on whether she was suicidally depressed or lacked adequate support systems. The judge also failed to note that almost all newly quadriplegic patients go through an initial period of depression and suicidal idealization. The judge claimed that his order would allow her to "die with dignity." A doctor, nurse, and respiratory therapist had to carry out the judge's order.

Ethical wars will also dictate health-care providers' rights of association. In the fall of 1998, Michigan voters defeated a physician-assisted suicide measure. The proposed measure would have prohibited hospitals, practices, nursing homes, and even associations from denying membership or privileges to health-care providers who participated in physician-assisted suicides. Nursing homes and hospitals would have been required to provide witnesses for patients signing requests for physician-assisted suicide on their premises. The measure would have also interfered with a doctor's rights to associate with the doctor's own patients.[4]

3. Mike Schneider, "Shooting Victim Dies," Associated Press story on ABC News.com (May 19, 1999). http://204.202.137.110/sections/us/DailyNews/righttodie990518.html

4. Consider this scenario: A doctor diagnoses metastatic breast cancer and estimates that the woman, a patient of the doctor for over twenty years, will live only a few months. On the next visit, the woman asks about physician-assisted suicide, which the doctor op-

More ethical fallout is on the way — evil practices always spread and worsen corruption. Just as abortion has led to the horror of partial-birth abortion, legalized physician-assisted suicide would corrupt the medical profession. Oregon's law requires doctors to lie on death certificates by forbidding them to list suicide as the cause of death. Through such deception, physician-assisted suicide requires insurance companies to invalidate their suicide exception clauses. It drops a shroud of secrecy around a profession that is built on trust engendered by open peer review.

Ultimately, the culture of death will corrupt the whole health-care system and destroy the foundation of trust. This is already beginning to occur in Holland, where fearful citizens carry cards saying, "Please don't euthanize me" in case of hospital admission. Some hire "sitters" to protect them from being euthanized against their will during their admission.

Along with new ethical standards will come the pressure to conform. Abortion advocates recently engineered a resolution by the American Medical Student Association calling for a formal requirement for abortion training on all medical school campuses. A few years ago, the American College of Graduate Medical Education tried to require abortion training for all residencies in obstetrics and gynecology. Subtle discrimination occurs in medical school and residency admissions on the basis of prospective students' moral and religious beliefs.[5]

Inhibitions

Clearly the outcome of the ethical wars will have a profound influence on individual health-care practitioners, their professions, and the health-care system. It is in every provider's interest to become involved before it is too late to affect the outcome. Yet, many do not. What inhibitions must be overcome to get caregivers — with all their knowledge, experience, and influence — *involved?*

---

poses on moral grounds. Under penalty of the law proposed in Michigan, the doctor is required immediately to transfer the patient and her records to a doctor who will help her kill herself. The doctor is given no room to try to dissuade the patient, treat her for any underlying depression, or even refer her to a psychiatrist for evaluation. Once she makes the request that conflicts with the doctor's ethics, the doctor is no longer allowed to associate with the patient.

5. This is done subtly — for instance, by asking candidates how they would handle a sixteen-year-old unmarried female with an eight-week pregnancy. Candidates who fail to offer abortion are likely to be eliminated from the admission list.

Many caregivers feel inhibited simply because they have not invested the time to consider ethical issues and establish personal positions. A health-care giver faces enormous time constraints, making it difficult to keep up in one's own field, much less make an impact as one proficient in bioethics.[6] Lack of time limits a caregiver's ability to develop a high-impact presentation necessary to influence his or her colleagues. Preparing these tools requires hours of research and documentation. Consumed by the demands of daily life and practice, many health-care professionals conclude that "sufficient today are the problems thereof." They do not recognize the consequences of changing the principles that have guided medicine for more than a millennium.

Some actually have blindly accepted the world's attitude of relativity. "What is right for you is right for you and what is right for me is right for me." Having elevated tolerance to the status of the primary virtue, they are reluctant to establish any position that requires a principled stance.

Those who take traditional positions on bioethics are sometimes unwilling or unable to communicate with or convince others. They are often hindered by a lack of knowledge on the issues. Doctors, nurses, and other caregivers are seen as professionals with credibility built upon their expertise. If they don't feel like experts on abortion, they may avoid opportunities to influence others on the issue.

Many health-care givers are inhibited by a real or perceived fear of the professional consequences of speaking out on ethical issues — particularly the no-compromise abortion issue. Health-care professionals, especially newcomers, who take a bold stand, are often discriminated against in salary, promotion, and job security.

Health-care providers are also concerned about speaking from the right platforms. To gain appropriate forums and be identified as a health-care professional, they must be positioned correctly before the church, media, public, and their colleagues.[7]

---

6. Increasing paperwork, seeing more patients in less time, and becoming an employee subject to the schedules of others make it difficult for doctors to find the time. Nurses' schedules are not much better, and the stress of their jobs has dramatically increased. They are expected to get more done with fewer trained personnel. Time constraints are a significant inhibitor to caregivers making a difference in the ethical wars.

7. As I stood on the steps of the Supreme Court the day physician-assisted suicide was argued, I had the opportunity to speak to many, but later realized that I would have had many more opportunities to influence public opinion if I had worn a white coat. The coat would have made me the only identifiable doctor present and attracted the hordes of media. Clearly identifying myself as a doctor would have given me the important platforms I sought as Executive Director of CMDS.

Strategy

Without the unity of a strategy, health-care professionals are also inhibited. A strategy brings clarity, explaining why they need to be involved and how their work can provide synergy for the entire effort. They must see a reasonable chance of winning the battle. Caregivers are accustomed to teamwork, drawing strength and focus within a group. Even a surgeon cannot do a major operation alone. A strategy requires leadership that calls for involvement, communicates the strategy, demonstrates by example, and continues to motivate, train, and equip those involved. As history proves, good leadership and logistics win battles.

On a practical level, how can a health-care provider's inhibitions be overcome? How can medical professionals be mobilized to make a greater difference in the days ahead?

Motivate

The first task is *motivation*. The leaders must sound the alarm and paint a clear picture of the implications to health-care provider and patient relationships. Use informational and emotive methods through direct mail, audiovisual presentations, meetings, and articles. Leaders must motivate not only Christian professionals, but also their colleagues in secular professional organizations.[8]

8. Last year CMDS contributed a lecture on physician-assisted suicide to an audio digest received by thousands of family practitioners. After hearing a very pro-assisted suicide lecture on this audio digest, I had kindly but firmly chastised the publisher of the audio magazine for failing to present a balanced view. I did not get a response for almost two months and thought he had disregarded my comments. Then a letter arrived saying, "I have had your letter on my desk for a couple of months, and every day would look at it and try to justify in my mind our actions. I finally have decided that we can't. We were wrong to give such an unbalanced view. Would you know of someone who could present the other side of the debate?" Realizing that time was of the essence, I walked into the CMDS studio and gave a lecture, sending it to the publisher. I did not hear anything for six months and had almost forgotten the incident. Then, one morning, I popped my latest Family Practice Audio Digest tape into my car tape deck as I headed to work. I almost had a wreck. I was the first speaker! That experience emboldened me last fall to explore how this material could get on the agenda at the American Academy of Family Practice (AAFP) 1999 annual meeting. After contacting the right person, who turned out to be a believer, I sent him the audio tape and some other materials. This led to my invitation to give the critical issue plenary on physician-assisted suicide at the national AAFP meeting. Did this happen because of my great talents or connections? No. It happened because I was motivated to sound the alarm.

Educate

The second strategy to overcome inhibitions is to *educate health-care givers.* Educational opportunities must emphasize practicality, quality, and convenient learning. Most caregivers do not have time to earn advanced degrees. But many are eager to get education that will enable them to make wise decisions in their practices and to influence others. CMDS and The Center for Bioethics and Human Dignity have co-sponsored "Breathtaking Decisions" conferences across the country. Informal educational techniques must also be utilized. Audiocassettes are a popular format for CMDS members. The Internet is quickly becoming the classroom of the future, with chat rooms gaining popularity and list servers catering to busy professionals.

Health-care providers must not only receive information but also learn how to use it effectively. *How* to communicate is as important as *what* to communicate. With that assumption, CMDS designed the resource kits "The Battle for Life" on physician-assisted suicide and "The Gift of Life" on abortion.[9] Each kit contains the interactive resources and materials to make any health-care professional an expert and to enable him or her to share the essential information.

CMDS conducted an educational campaign on physician-assisted suicide before the Michigan referendum in the fall of 1998. Throughout my statewide speaking tour, students and professionals requested the information I had displayed in a well-documented PowerPoint presentation. By placing it on our web site (www.cmds.org), CMDS allowed them to download, modify, and use the presentation. We want to empower our allies in the battle.

Unify

The raging ethical battles require a unified strategy and coordination. This increases the chances of success, avoids duplicating effort, and is most cost-effective. Major donors are attracted to joint efforts and clear strategies. The

9. The abortion kit contains books, pamphlets, pictures, a video, speaker's notes, handouts, biblical and secular references, a bulletin insert that can be copied, and more. By purchasing items in bulk, we passed on savings to our members. We have sold thousands of these all-in-one resources to educate purchasers and provide them with the tools to influence others. We are currently providing an interactive CD on genetics and human cloning, which will contain over 100 PowerPoint slides, audio interviews, handouts, and other resources. To order an educational kit, call 1-888-231-2637.

expense of major campaigns does not preclude the involvement of groups like CMDS, Nurses Christian Fellowship, Christian Pharmacy Fellowship, and the Christian Legal Society. These organizations have the influence of memberships, an impressive and effective source of strength. A membership of thousands far outweighs a mailing list of tens of thousands. These smaller groups can also highly leverage their efforts and do a lot at a low cost. By motivating and educating members, CMDS impacted the Michigan physician-assisted suicide battle of 1998 for a total cost of under $10,000.

Through mailings and a statewide speaking tour, doctors were encouraged to educate their patients. They were given materials to place in examining rooms and a sample letter to write to their patients. This letter explained why they opposed the legalization of physician-assisted suicide and would never participate in providing it. Patients valued the professional perspective of their personal physicians, and the mailings strengthened the patient-doctor bond.

CMDS also encouraged doctors to leverage their influence through community organizations, such as Rotary and Lions clubs, and professional forums, including county medical societies and hospital grand rounds. We developed a statewide speakers bureau for media interviews and appearances on radio and television.

Church involvement is key to the battle on physician-assisted suicide. Lack of church involvement may have contributed to the Oregon defeat. In Michigan, CMDS contacted churches across the state with a mailing to alert them to the issue and to make speakers available. The churches created greater demand for speakers than could be met by our speakers bureau! To meet this need, only four weeks before the referendum vote, we produced a 25-minute video for less than $2 per tape. We distributed the videos to more than 500 churches, reaching an estimated 100,000 viewers. That is cost-effective leverage!

In public awareness campaigns, use proven methods to change opinions. This requires polling, focus groups, professional marketing firms, and a savvy use of the media. Since mainstream radio and TV advertising was cost prohibitive, CMDS leveraged assets through a video news release. Two media staff persons interviewed key CMDS members involved in end-of-life care along with terminally ill patients who were opposed to physician-assisted suicide. The two-minute video releases were shown on 84 percent of the 47 television stations that received them. For approximately $1,500 total cost, the CMDS message impacted millions of prime-time viewers through compelling patient interviews.

Throughout the Michigan campaign, the CMDS national office continued to produce late-breaking news releases and provide dozens of TV, radio, and print interviews representing our membership. As a smaller organization, we could quickly change directions, martial our staff, and respond.

Leadership

To win wars, good leadership is the key. Leaders must lead from the front by example. They must be willing to expose themselves to the greatest danger and to clearly address the issues. People follow people. They are looking for leaders to articulate their heartfelt concerns, to teach them and lead them into battle.

Each of us has our own sphere of influence. Although the tools CMDS has used may not be available to you, the strategies and principles hold true. Leadership is needed now more than ever before.

God uses people like Moses who feared he could not speak well enough. God uses people like Gideon who complained that he was the "least in the family," and even headstrong, uneducated fishermen like Peter. God does not necessarily call those already equipped. He equips the called for the task ahead.

Christian health-care providers are the leadership in Christian bioethics. Each individual and organization must band together to motivate, train, and equip health-care professionals and the public. With intellect and influence, we can make a vital difference in the ethical wars that lie ahead.

A Call to Moral Leadership

Barbara J. White, R.N., Ed.D.

As Dr. David Stevens has wisely and accurately stated, Christian health-care professionals have a unique platform from which to speak and act as we face the moral dilemmas in today's world. I, too, believe that God has placed us in health-care positions for just such a time as this, to be a moral conscience, to speak the truth, and to make a life-affirming impact on our culture. We are called to moral leadership.

The upheaval in the health-care industry has created unprecedented ethical dilemmas, ambiguity, and moral tension. In a world of accelerating change, health-care reform has resulted in fundamental changes throughout the system. In response to the need to control health-care costs, managed care is now the predominate form of health-care delivery. The business of health care has created market-share competition and for-profit corporate entities. In the midst of these changes, the moral obligations of health-care professionals and organizations are in flux.

At the same time that we are concerned about allocation of limited resources and cost constraints, advanced technology scientists continue to unravel the complex strands of DNA, gene therapy is being used for diseases, and cloning is no longer science fiction but reality. Ethical issues such as embryo engineering, selective reduction, partial birth abortion, futile care, assisted suicide, and rationing create unprecedented conflict. In the midst of these changes, the moral rights and duties of individuals and health-care providers are in disarray.

We are in a moral crisis in health care today, a crisis that has more to do with values than with economics. Medicine and nursing are scientific, practice-based disciplines, but they are also moral endeavors concerned with human decency. Our moral work involves intimate relationship with vulnerable human beings. Yet conflicting values and shifting parameters make it increasingly difficult to find a common moral purpose. More and more members of the health-care community no longer agree on universal principles. The result is that many health-care providers lack the surety of an accurate compass to guide them through these challenging and difficult times. As Christians, we have a moral compass. Scripture provides the principles and prayer and the Holy Spirit provide the guidance as we face the obstacles. The issue is really one of willingness to act on our beliefs.

In my role as nursing faculty, I have the privilege of teaching students about the nursing profession. The joys of teaching are many, but one of the greatest rewards is to encourage students to give voice to their beliefs and then to see them live out their convictions. One student in particular, who graduated with her nursing degree a year ago in May, is already influencing nursing as a moral leader. Jessica is twenty-three years old. She is intelligent, competent, compassionate, highly motivated, and articulate. During school, she became involved in Nurses Christian Fellowship (NCF) and began to grow in her relationship with the Lord. In her words, her faith became a heart matter, not just head knowledge. Since graduation, I have had the opportunity to mentor Jessica, to disciple her, to encourage her, and to pray with her about critical issues in practice. She works on a very busy oncology unit in a large acute care hospital. One day as a new graduate, she had an especially heavy patient assignment. She administered over twenty intravenous medications including potassium and blood, and she was involved in a medication error incident. As she sat before the risk manager and the quality review board of the hospital in fear for her job, we prayed specifically that God would give her the courage to speak the truth about the real issues. As system procedures and protocols were discussed and reviewed, Jessica stood firm on her convictions. Yes, some system changes would be beneficial, but the real issues of patient load and R.N. staffing needed to be addressed. Jessica did not lose her job that day. There were other battles for her to fight. On her unit, many patients in severe pain are offered relief through narcotic drips. According to Jessica, some nurses prefer to place patients on a continuous drip to save time instead of medicating the patient frequently in small amounts to prevent over-sedation and premature death. She disagrees with this practice and tells this story:

> Last week I had a dying man under my care that begged me not to give him anything that would make him sleep. He was terrified of not waking up. His physician ordered medication to calm him, control his pain, and poten-

tially lead to his death. I firmly refused to give the medication and reminded the physician that, if given, he might die five minutes later. The physician replied that, if not given, he would die of exhaustion. I told her that I would not give it, even if it meant he was exhausted. He wanted to be with his family. God would take him when he was ready. Instead, I prayed with him. Amazingly enough, God and I were able to keep his pain under control. The patient lived for a few more days and even made it home under hospice care.

As a young new graduate in nursing, Jessica is living out her convictions. Jessica is heeding the call to moral leadership in today's health-care arena.

Over this past year, I have also had the privilege of interviewing several nurse executives in large corporate hospitals. We have talked about the meaning of moral leadership in today's health-care environment, the dilemmas that these nurse leaders face within their institutions, and the values that prevail as they resolve moral dilemmas. Before beginning this research, I believed that the ethic of care was being eroded by an overall concern for cost and that the ethic of patient advocacy was being replaced by the ethic of stewardship of resources. I have not found this to be true. Instead, preliminary data analysis has revealed a strong basis for quality patient care. These nurse executives have learned to balance advocacy and stewardship, and to blend cost and caring. These are leaders with clear vision and strong values. They are people of influence who are willing to stand on convictions for the sake of patients and nursing staff. They are heeding their call to moral leadership. It was interesting that all of the nurse executives that I interviewed mentioned strong religious backgrounds and beliefs that provided the framework for their decision-making.

There is much opposition to the Christian worldview in our culture today. God's word tells us that moral leaders are developed and tested by opposition. Moral leaders must be more committed to courage than they are to comfort and complacency.

As I think about the moral leadership that is so desperately needed in health care today, I am reminded of another time millennia ago when moral chaos reigned. The biblical book of Esther tells of a time during Esther's life when there was a moral crisis that forced her to make a decision involving total commitment.[1] Esther was an orphan who, after the death of her parents, was raised by her older Jewish cousin, Mordecai. She grew into a young woman of extraordinary grace and beauty. She won the favor of everyone

---

1. Sid Buzzell, ed., *The Leadership Bible: Leadership Principles from God's Word* (Grand Rapids: Zondervan, 1998).

who saw her, including the Persian king Xerxes who selected Esther as his queen. Soon after, Haman, a sinister official in the court, developed a plot to execute all of the Jews in the Persian empire. In short, the messianic line was in danger of extinction. Mordecai begged Esther to go to the king to persuade him to call off the terrible plan.

Esther's initial response to Mordecai's plea was typical of those not wanting to get involved. Esther said that she had to follow protocol. She could not go before the king without being summoned. If she did, there was a good chance that she could lose her life. Why should she risk her life to persuade the king to change a decree? Why should anyone risk personal gain or position to help others?

Moral leadership demands that we speak up for what is right, and that we act on God's principles. We must serve others, and use our resources to rescue, to develop, to edify those under our charge. If we don't, who will? Mordecai had no sympathy for Esther's refusal to help. He was a man of commitment. Mordecai responded to Esther's refusal with three profound challenges that strike at the heart of Esther's reluctance.

- The first challenge repositioned Esther within the *conflict*. Esther was a Jew, too. The decree impacted her just as it impacted the rest of the Jewish nation. Mordecai stated: "Do not think that because you are in the king's house, you alone of all the Jews will escape." Don't let the comfort and security of your position hinder you from being involved. You cannot escape the situation. Your position places you within the conflict.
- The second challenge reminded Esther of her *call*. Esther had the privilege to perform, to speak and act on moral conviction. If she didn't act courageously and use her privilege wisely, she would be pushed aside and her role would be given to someone else. Mordecai said: "For if you remain silent at this time, relief and deliverance for the Jews will arise from another place. . . ." God is at work in this world. It is a privilege to respond to God's call.
- The third challenge required Esther to act on her *convictions*. Mordecai's counsel to Esther in 4:14 defines the essence of moral leadership and should be written boldly on every leader's heart and mind. "Who knows but that you have come to [your] position for such a time as this?" Each of us has unique gifts and influence to be used for God's glory.

In essence, Mordecai reminded Esther that God was sovereign and in charge. Esther was his servant. Her position of power and leadership was by his choice and for his purpose. I love Esther's response: it had a strategy that involved others and it was a heart response of total commitment. Esther called on her fellow believers to pray and fast. And then she cast herself, her very life, on God, in dependence on him. How did God work in the situation? Scripture tells us that the king's heart went out to Esther; that he extended his golden scepter; that Esther's life was spared; and that the Jewish people were gloriously rescued. In a culture in which women did not rule, Esther was a woman of enormous influence who saved her nation from extinction. Esther heeded her call to moral leadership.

Esther and all others who lead must view their gifts, their resources, even their very life, as God's tools for accomplishing his special plan. Our call to moral leadership is not without risk. Esther knew that she would take a life-threatening risk to appeal to the king on behalf of her people. My former student Jessica knew that she was risking her job to speak out on behalf of her patients. Some risk position, others risk power or prestige. What are you willing to risk?

Cassie Bernall, a victim in the Columbine High School shooting, risked it all. She lost her life to gain eternal reward.[2] Cassie's martyrdom is remarkable when you consider that it was just two years ago that she gave her heart to Jesus. Before that, she dabbled in the occult and witchcraft, and embraced the same darkness that drove her killers to this despicable act. When Cassie became a Christian, however, she dedicated her life to Christ, wholeheartedly and completely. She turned her life around and embraced a courageous faith.[3]

On the Sunday evening before her death, Cassie Bernall shared her testimony with her church family.[4] As we face the challenges in health care and as we work to plan effective strategies, Cassie becomes a sterling example in her conflict, in her calling, and in her commitment to her conviction.

We are in a moral crisis in health care today. We have a call from God to stand and act on moral convictions. My prayer for all of us is that we, like Cassie, Jessica, and Esther, will heed the call. Together, we can make a difference.

2. P. Hiett, *Making Sense: Reflections on Columbine High School,* Golden, Colo.: Lookout Mountain Community Church, April 25, 1999.

3. G. Kirsten, personal interview in July, 1999, at West Boales Community Church, Littleton, Colo.

4. Youth group tribute to Cassie Bernall, West Boales Community Church, Littleton, Colo., 1999; information from video used by permission.

Paradigm Lost?
New Techniques for Engagement
in Medical Education

Gregory W. Rutecki, M.D.

In 1 Timothy 4:12, Paul offers this advice, "Do not let anyone look down on you because you are young." In many ways, the previous generation has "looked down" on everything and everyone postmodern. There has been a stubborn refusal to recognize changing cultural tides. Opportunities provided for cross-generational evangelism between what have become disparate cultures invariably seem to reach an impasse. The all-too-common result is the misreading of an entire generation, with most participants failing to discern the absence of a common frame of reference. In reality, evangelism to postmodern people framed in a modernist perspective has become a bit like putting the new wine of the kingdom into old wineskins.

Charles Colson described such an impasse when he related the experience of having dinner with a media personality, a member of postmodern culture.[1] After describing his conversion, Mr. Colson was told in no uncertain terms by his dinner guest, "Obviously Jesus worked for you, crystals and channeling worked for my friend — just like your Jesus." Colson's attempt to explain Jesus' exclusivity reached that impasse again. Intriguingly, the Woody

---

1. C. Colson, "Reaching the Pagan Mind," *Christianity Today,* Nov. 9, 1992, p. 112.

I am indebted to Trinity International University, John Kilner, D. A. Carson, and Roger Lundin for many of the ideas in this manuscript defining postmodernism.

186

Allen movie "Crimes and Misdemeanors" — about a killer who extinguishes any sense of guilt with the conclusion that life is but survival of the fittest — captured the listener's interest. Then a discussion of moral law followed, touching on Tolstoy, C. S. Lewis, and the Bible and culminating in Christ's atoning sacrifice. Colson commented further: "My experience is a sobering illustration of how resistant the modern mind has become to the Christian message. And it raises serious questions about the effectiveness of traditional evangelistic methods in our age. For the spirit of the age is changing more quickly than many of us realize."[2]

G. E. Veith has observed that the consistent difficulty in engaging postmoderns has been in finding a common frame of reference.[3] "Usual" evangelistic approaches no longer work. The following discussion will chronicle my own efforts, one pilgrim's progress, to better understand Paul's message in 1 Corinthians 9:20-23 (NIV):

> To the Jews, I became like a Jew. . . . To those under the law, I became like one under the law. . . . To those not having the law, I became like one not having the law. . . . To the weak, I became weak. . . . I have become all things to all men so that by all possible means I might save some. I do this all for the sake of the gospel. . . .

One Physician's Primer on Postmodern Culture

"If modernism represented a desperate effort to have art and culture fill the void created by the decline of religion in the west, then postmodernism stands as the affirmation of the void, as the declaration of the impossibility of ever filling it."[4]

Before proceeding further, fundamental definitions are necessary, especially for the words "culture" and "postmodernism." The definitions will be followed by the vocabulary and unique identifiers of postmodern culture, including the so-called mistrust of metanarratives, the process of deconstruction, and the important descriptor, a "culture of interpretation."

Kevin Vanhoozer has defined culture and postmodernism incisively both by words and by metaphor.

2. Colson, "Reaching the Pagan Mind."

3. G. E. Veith Jr., *Postmodern Times: A Christian Guide to Contemporary Thought and Culture* (Wheaton, Ill.: Crossway Books, 1994), pp. 15-16.

4. R. Lundin, *The Culture of Interpretation: Christian Faith and the Postmodern World* (Grand Rapids: Eerdmans, 1993), pp. 3-4.

Culture may be defined as the objectification, the expression in words and works of the "spirit" of a particular people who inhabit a particular time and place. Culture is the effort of the human spirit to express itself by building and embodying values and beliefs into concrete forms. . . . Culture expresses the totality of what a group of humans value. . . . It expresses who we are and why we are valuable.[5]

For those who like to conceptualize from metaphor, Vanhoozer's description of culture, drawing from Shakespeare, is invaluable.[6] He begins with the quote, "All the world's a stage" from the play "As You Like It." He observes further that medieval morality plays were performed on three separate stages: the middle stage was earth with God observing from a superior vantage point and Satan from an inferior one. He then offers important advice: "As Christians, if life is indeed a stage, we have the ultimate set of stage directions in God's word. It is our job to discover and articulate a way of wisdom to our culture."[7] In this important metaphorical context, culture is a "performance" of one's ultimate beliefs and values, a concrete way of staging one's "religion."

Individuals are actors and actresses, but they are culturally and historically costumed and thrown into plots that are culturally and historically conditioned. They may not be given particular lines, but they are given a particular language. Culture is the scenery, the environment, the world into which one is thrown when one appears on stage. If the world is a stage, culture provides the props that fill it.[8]

Indeed, if postmodern culture does not provide specific lines, it does provide a language. The foundation for that language begins with a skepticism towards metanarratives. Postmoderns feel free to see themselves as neither defined nor confined by the historical or communal narratives that make claims upon them.[9] For example, the authority of the Bible or of the multiple volumes of Western literature is considered to be no more than a mask for a "will to power." They have been replaced by postmoderns' radical interpretation of history.

For instance, during the 1987-1988 school year, Stanford University es-

---

5. K. J. Vanhoozer, "The World Well Staged?" in *God and Culture,* ed. D. A. Carson and John D. Woodbridge (Grand Rapids: Eerdmans, 1993), p. 2.

6. Vanhoozer, "The World Well Staged?" pp. 1-30.

7. Vanhoozer, "The World Well Staged?" p. 2.

8. Vanhoozer, "The World Well Staged?" p. 2.

9. Lundin, *Culture of Interpretation,* p. 6.

sentially dismantled its Western civilization curriculum.[10] The committee taking that action felt that the European tradition was in place to "perpetuate racist and sexist stereotypes and to reinforce notions of cultural superiority that are wounding to some and dangerous to all in a world of such evident diversity."[11] Contained within this mistrust of metanarratives is the notion that a "core list" of readings is inherently flawed and creates only the illusion of an absolute or universal human history. Thus, for example, Shakespeare's King Lear is no longer a father mistreated by his daughters, but rather a character from a story concerning radical feminists who rebel against an inherently flawed patriarchal structure.

Furthermore, for postmoderns, all traditional and religious literature should undergo a "deconstruction." Since postmoderns believe that truth cannot be known, writings must be taken apart and meaning must be "reconstructed" by a culture that establishes its own "truth." What is left should be replaced by a radical hermeneutic characterized by an individual's perspective, a primacy of subjectivity, and an affirmation of the resultant chaos. Thus, postmoderns inhabit a culture of their own interpretation.

Flowing from these definitions is a language that cannot render truths about the world in an objective way, but rather language as cultural creation. Word meanings have become merely a social construct. The result is an increasing variety of neologisms such as the word "open-mindedness," which is no longer connected with the willingness to consider alternative views, but rather is associated with a dogmatic relativizing of all views.[12] A radical hermeneutic also affects movies — the new narratives of postmodernism. The movie version of "The Scarlet Letter" ends without the Christian message of repentance. It is replaced by Hester and Arthur Dimmesdale living happily ever after without a sense of guilt for adultery.[13] The infinite variations and relativizing of words has led to a postmodern Babel, with language reduced to each individual's personal interpretation.

Paradigm Lost: A New One Provided

Last year, the Bannockburn Institute sponsored a symposium to equip attendees with evangelistic techniques aimed at postmodern culture. Evangelists to

10. Lundin, *Culture of Interpretation,* pp. 19ff.
11. Lundin, *Culture of Interpretation,* p. 23.
12. D. A. Carson, "Christian Witness in an Age of Pluralism," in *God and Culture,* p. 34.
13. Lundin, *Culture of Interpretation,* pp. 137ff.

postmoderns from disparate settings — pastors from Europe, professors at secular and Christian universities, college chaplains, to name a few — shared their experiences in bridging that aforementioned impasse between cultures. A sample of titles included: "An ancient message with modern means to a postmodern mind" by Ravi Zacharias; "Communicating sin in a postmodern world" by Mark Dever; "Finding God at Harvard: Reaching the post-Christian university" by Kelly Monroe; and "Penetrating ethnic pluralism" by Charles Gilmer.[14] The conference awoke many from both spiritual and dogmatic slumbers and made alive Paul's imperative in Romans 13:11 to understand the present age. The course ended with a challenge. D. A. Carson observed,

> At another level we are returning, through no virtue of our own, to something analogous to the pluralistic world the earliest Christians had to confront, and so in this sense the New Testament can be applied to us and our culture more directly than was possible fifty years ago. Christian witness has become a matter of confronting a bewildering variety of worldview perspectives with the Bible's story and with the Gospel as its crowning point. Though we are faced with a bewildering array of beliefs — crystals, channeling, syncretic religions, to name but a few — we must remember that early Christians encountered people who worshipped rocks, believed plants could be deities, sacrificed animals, accepted ritual castration and prostitution.[15]

For example, a professor from a secular university has discovered a common frame of reference with postmoderns through "Crimes and Misdemeanors," a movie already mentioned. In it a married ophthalmologist carries on an affair until his mistress threatens to tell his wife. He hires someone to kill his mistress and, after initially experiencing guilt, decides his response should be emblematic of survival of the fittest. He goes on with life, free of any of the encumbrances Dostoevsky's guilt-ridden Raskalnikov experienced. During the ensuing discussion, postmoderns may be asked whether they can be comfortable in a world that does not experience guilt. Spirited discussion often follows concerning contemporary nihilism — a result of subjectivity and the relativization of truth portrayed in the movie.

One pastor, who consistently encounters postmodern "seekers" at his church, has utilized biblical sermons portraying God as a feeling and in-

---

14. From the Bannockburn Institute for Christianity and Contemporary Culture, Telling the Truth: Evangelizing Postmoderns Series, 1998.

15. See Carson, *God and Culture,* pp. 44-45. See also D. A. Carson, *Athens Revisited: Evangelizing Biblical Illiterates,* in the Telling the Truth: Evangelizing Postmoderns Series, 1998.

tensely emotional being.[16] Postmoderns have a mistrust of rational explanations and theories. They prefer emotionalism and feeling, particularly trusting subjectivity in the acquisition of truth. So, as an example, this pastor preaches from Hosea 11:1-11, portraying God's tender nostalgia, apparent as God teaches Ephraim to walk, as he leads with cords of human kindness and with ties of love. Such an approach remains true to the scriptural text while at the same time providing that common frame of reference.

One can extrapolate this culturally sensitive method of evangelism to a different audience: that of medical students and residents in a postmodern environment. As Ravi Zacharias has implored, all must discover points of contact in a desensitized culture. Who needs this sensitivity and contact more than young physicians entrusted with those bearing the image of God?

A New Paradigm Applied to Medical Education

Understanding that the focus has switched from metanarratives to movies and other mass media permits educators to select similar vehicles that engender discussion about essential ethical topics. For medicine, justice in both research and allocation decisions is an important topic. In that context, May of 1999 marked an event worth noting.[17]

May 14, 1999, was the anniversary of President Clinton's formal apology for the Tuskegee Study. In the study, the U.S. Public Health Service followed 399 African American males with syphilis without informed consent or treatment. Also, during the same month, the Office for Protection from Research Risks charged Duke University's Institutional Review Board with insufficient administrative oversight of human studies and violation of federal conflict of interest rules. Thus, it appears that justice needs further articulation in the specific arena of human research.

There is a well-done HBO movie entitled "Miss Ever's Boys," which chronicles the Tuskegee experiment. A two-hour bioethics session has been allotted in the curriculum to show the movie. Even though the movie exceeded the time allotment, the students refused to leave until the movie was finished. At the next discussion session, the students were asked to design an experiment for a drug named pimagedine, an agent that may prevent the

---

16. Roy Clements, *The Passion at the Heart of the Universe*, in the Telling the Truth: Evangelizing Postmoderns Series, 1998.

17. J. Ellis, "Alleged Safety and Ethics Violations Prompt Careful Review of Clinical Trials," *Academic Physician & Scientist*, July/August 1999, p. 1.

complications of diabetes. However, pimagedine is a double-edged sword associated with significant complications. The students were asked to design experiments from rats to humans in order to "come to grips" so to speak with the purpose of an Institutional Review Board and a Safety Monitoring Committee. They had to retain the scientific rigor necessary for a double-blind study without harming their subjects, sequentially administering the medication to healthy and eventually ill individuals with diabetes. They were even asked how much money to give to indigent patients to enroll in the study without financially manipulating them. Despite a prevailing postmodern mindset, justice appeared to be vindicated in their final design. They were all disturbed about potential future Tuskegee experiments.

Dr. John Kilner and I have been privileged to write a paper for *Seminars in Dialysis* regarding justice in the context of dialysis rationing.[18] The conclusion was that the only just way to ration was through a lottery. A lottery obviates society's fallenness displayed in prior allocation decisions — a fallenness demonstrating racial, age, and gender bias. In fact, dialysis is often chosen as an allocation paradigm since early access was strictly rationed. Prior to Medicare funding for dialysis, there were more patients than machines. Analysis of those allocation decisions in the 1960s and 1970s demonstrated that minorities, the elderly, and women were dialyzed less often. Limitation of resources in certain areas since then (for example, solid organ transplantation) has shown that the bias has not changed.

In order to engage postmoderns, when the results of the paper are presented, limited dialysis stations can be compared to too few lifeboats on *The Titanic*. The immense popularity of the movie ensures that virtually all postmoderns are familiar with the details. Lifeboats were prioritized based on social value — the rich got richer, and the poor, ultimately "poorer." The audience identifies with this analogy and starts to realize that a lottery is not so extreme after all. God himself is no respecter of persons. The correlation between the movie and dialysis access provides that important common frame of reference.

Whither Goes the Bible?

There is also a context for the Bible in postmodern environments. An opportunity arose from a short story by Richard Selzer, a prolific physician-writer.

---

18. G. W. Rutecki and J. Kilner, "Dialysis as a Resource Allocation Paradigm: Confronting Tragic Choices Once Again?" *Seminars in Dialysis* 12 (1999): 38-43.

He has written a story about transplant donation entitled, "Whither Thou Goest"[19] which essentially is organ transplantation as metaphor, utilizing the story of Ruth from the Old Testament. The story itself is only twenty-one pages long and quite readable. In it, the wife Hannah donates her husband Sam's organs after he is shot to death acting as a Good Samaritan. She cannot come to closure after he dies and face the rest of her life until she listens to his heart again — albeit in the chest of the recipient. This short story engages a number of concepts including *hesed* or God's lovingkindness, which is mirrored in the donation of organs. It also encounters the hope of resurrection; and it applies the metaphor of harvesting wheat or "gleaning" for organ donation.

There is also a sexual connotation in the story true to Ruth's encounter with Boaz on the threshing floor (Ruth 3:1-18). The gentleman with Sam's heart in his chest is taken aback to learn that Hannah wants to "auscultate" without a stethoscope! Students can be reminded that Rene Lannaec invented the stethoscope to avoid ear to chest auscultation in young females. The entire story and discussion presents the Bible as important literature in a medical context.

Also, I recently wrote a paper that scientifically explicated the Numbers 11 incident from the Old Testament, which describes the Israelites' apparent poisoning by quail.[20] In reality, the event is the first description of a syndrome named rhabdomyolysis and substantiates the truth of Scripture. Rhabdomyolysis is severe muscle injury with the leakage of muscle contents into the circulation. Complications include kidney failure (called myoglobinuric renal failure) and death from respiratory muscle paralysis. The risk factors for rhabdomyolysis incurred by quail ingestion, described during the twentieth century, include muscular exertion by the ingestees, the specific species of spring migratory quail indigenous to the Middle East, and fresh quail ingested soon after capture — were all present as the event was described in Scripture. Numbers 11 is the first description of this disease, is medically accurate, and is referenced as such in major contemporary reviews of myoglobinuric renal failure.[21]

19. R. Selzer, "Whither Thou Goest," in *Imagine a Woman and Other Tales* (Lansing: Michigan State University Press, 1996), pp. 1-21.

20. G. W. Rutecki, J. D. Geib, and A. Ognibene, "Rhabdomyolysis in Antiquity: From Ancient Descriptions to Scientific Explication," *The Pharos of Alpha Omega Alpha* 61 (1998): 18-22.

21. R. Zager, "Rhabdomyolysis and Myohemoglobinuric Acute Renal Failure," *Kid. Int.* 49 (1996): 314-26.

A Paradox Found:
Medicine as the Most Scientific of the Humanities

Despite their postmodern heritage, medical students are forced to be scientific and can often be engaged in scientific discussions that have religious ramifications. A classic example is the evolution versus intelligent design debate. The book by Michael Behe, *Darwin's Black Box,*[22] can be utilized in discussions that allow engagement of postmodern students with or without religious backgrounds. These discussions can serve as outreach for Christian Medical & Dental Society groups. Classic organs and mechanisms that fit well into the intelligent design format are the eye, the hemoglobin molecule, and the blood-clotting cascade.

Transparencies of eye structures (the cornea, lens, retina, the aqueous and vitreous humors) can be utilized to demonstrate that random mutations are hard-pressed to explain eye function. The eye is an all-or-none organ and any one design flaw (blood vessels in the lens or humors, a lack of coordination with the occipital cortex) would render the organ essentially useless. The same can be said for hemoglobin wherein twenty-plus amino acids must be coordinated or the entire molecule is nonfunctional. Blood clotting is also complex enough to suggest intelligent design. The interplay of pro- and anti-coagulants (prothrombin and protein C for example) and the number of proteins in the intrinsic and extrinsic pathways may be utilized to suggest design.

These sessions allow the CMDS group to be outward rather than inward focused. They also permit medical students to see that Christian physicians do not surrender their scientific acumen.

Encounters with Postmodernism Serve as a Reminder of Acts 17:16-34

Like Paul's contemporaries, we inhabit a culture "full of idols"[23] (Acts 17:16) who might perceive our description of the resurrection as akin to being "babblers of strange ideas" (Acts 17:18). But since postmodern culture is very "religious," we have a phenomenal opportunity to lead its inhabitants through movies, short stories, and intelligent design discussions from their unknown

22. M. Behe, *Darwin's Black Box: The Biochemical Challenge to Evolution* (New York: The Free Press, 1996).

23. Carson, *God and Culture,* p. 45, and *Athens Revisited: Evangelizing Biblical Illiterates.*

god to the story which culminates in the gospel. At each moment, especially in the medical field, we must mirror the example of the great healer. Our compassion at the bedside characterized by a covenantal model of care goes a long way in engaging their interest, curiosity, and respect. The manner in which we approach the widow, the indigent, and the least of these brethren is not lost on those we teach. We cannot be reminded and encouraged too often that despite the fact that cultures change, Jesus Christ is the same yesterday, today, and forever.

Disability and Its Interdisciplinary Implications

Linda L. Treloar, R.N., Ph.D.

After developing an incomplete spinal cord injury following an accident in which a truck hit the tractor he was driving, 29-year-old Jim moved from visible physical disability and paralysis to a world where disability continues but a wheelchair is no longer required. Jim says:

> You know it's really weird. In some ways it's hard to enter into that wheelchair life, to go into that life and then come back out of it again. I entered into a whole other realm [life with paralysis] that I'd only observed. I stepped into the unknown and pulled back out of it again. Yet, one foot is still in that world.[1]

According to Jim, disability may create a "whole other realm," an "unknown" world. Despite our best intentions, health professionals may lack awareness of the divergence of perceptual worlds created by disability, and of the historical, sociopolitical context, and culture that surrounds disability. Although I am a nurse and the parent of a young adult with disabilities, I had much to learn about the perspectives of people affected by disability. Regardless of your experience or familiarity with disability, I urge you to seriously consider the question posed to me: "You're not disabled, how can you understand disability?"

---

1. All quotations from people affected by disabilities are published in: Linda L. Treloar, "Perceptions of Spiritual Beliefs, Response to Disability, and the Church" (doctoral dissertation, The Union Institute, Cincinnati, OH), in *Dissertation Abstracts International,* vol./issue 60-02A (University Microfilms International No. AAI9919753) (1999).

This essay describes clinical applications for health-care practice with people who have disabilities and their family members. It provides illustrations from qualitative research that explored connections between the spiritual beliefs of people affected by disability and their responses to living with disability.[2] I conducted unstructured conversational interviews with thirty persons affected by disability who lived in a metropolitan area in the Southwest during 1998. The participants included two major groups: nine adults with physical disabilities and thirteen parents of children with mixed developmental disabilities. Eight family members and other participants provided additional data. The participants ascribed to evangelical Christian beliefs and acknowledged a belief in the Bible as the inspired, inerrant, authoritative Word of God. I utilized grounded theory methods for coding and analysis of transcribed data.[3]

I use the participants' voices to stimulate the reader's understanding of disability, rather than to report the findings of the study per se. I discuss practical applications for multidisciplinary health professionals based on themes from the data.

Context for Disability, Spirituality, and Health

Both the Rehabilitation Act of 1973 (Section 504) and the Americans with Disabilities Act of 1990 use three descriptors to define disability. These include a physical or mental impairment that substantially limits one or more major life activities of an individual, a person with a record of such impairment, or a person who is regarded as having such an impairment.[4] A *major life activity* includes the ability to breathe, walk, see, hear, speak, work, care for oneself, perform manual tasks, and learn.[5] Physical disabilities, learning disabilities, intellectual disabilities, serious emotional disturbances, and health problems such as AIDS and asthma are examples of disabilities that may *substantially limit at least one major life activity.*

According to The International Classification of Impairments, Disabil-

2. Ibid.

3. Barney G. Glaser, *Basics of Grounded Theory Analysis: Emergence versus Forcing* (Mill Valley, Calif.: Sociology Press, 1992); Glaser, *Theoretical Sensitivity* (Mill Valley, Calif.: Sociology Press, 1978).

4. U.S. Department of Justice, "A Guide to Disability Rights Laws" (Pueblo, Colo.: Consumer Information Center, 1996).

5. Paul Wehman, ed., *The ADA Mandate for Social Change* (Baltimore, Md.: Paul H. Brookes, 1993).

ities, and Handicaps (ICIDH), a *disability* involves any restriction on or lack of ability to perform an activity in that manner or within the range considered normal.[6] An anatomical, mental, or psychological loss or another abnormality is an *impairment*. A *handicap* is a disadvantage resulting from impairment or disability.

Our feelings and thoughts about disability may conjure up conflicts between weakness and strength, dependency and independence, difficulty and heroism. We prefer to think that disability happens to "the other person." Yet nearly one in every five persons, 54 million people in the United States, has a disabling condition that interferes with life activities.[7]

Language and attitudes surrounding disability reveal centuries-old beliefs involving stereotype, stigma, and devaluation.[8] Johnson and Johnson coined the word "disaphobia" to describe the "prejudice, ignorance, fear and anxiety that persons feel in their interaction with the disabled, based on societal stigmatization."[9] Murphy, an anthropologist, reports in *The Body Silent:*

> One cannot . . . shelve a disability or hide it from the world. A serious disability inundates all other claims to social standing. . . . It is not a role; it is an identity, a dominant characteristic to which all social roles must be adjusted. And just as the paralytic cannot clear his mind of his impairment, society will not let him forget it.
>
> This one obvious fact, the disabled person's radical bodily difference, his departure from the human standard, dominates the thoughts of the other and may even repel him. But these are thoughts that can barely be articulated, let alone voiced.
>
> The disabled are more than deviants. They are the antiphony of everyday life. Just as the bodies of the disabled are permanently impaired, so also is their standing as members of society. . . . Their persons are regarded as contaminated; eyes are averted and people take care not to approach wheel-

6. Andrew M. Pope and Alvin R. Tarlov, eds., *Disability in America: Toward a National Agenda for Prevention* (Washington, D.C.: National Academy Press, 1991).

7. National Organization on Disability/Louis Harris and Associates, *N.O.D./Harris 1998 Survey of Americans with Disabilities* [electronic] (online: http://www.nod.org/presssurvey.html, accessed July 23, 1998).

8. Alan Gartner and Tom Joe, eds., *Images of the Disabled, Disabling Images* (New York: Praeger, 1987); Paul K. Longmore, "Uncovering the Hidden History of People with Disabilities," *Reviews in American History* 15, no. 3 (1987): 355-64.

9. Allen F. Johnson and Lori S. Johnson, "Shame and Spirituality: Taboo Topics in the Disability Community," *Journal of Religion in Disability and Rehabilitation* 2, no. 3 (1995): 31.

chairs too closely. My colleague Jessica Scheer refers to wheelchairs as "portable seclusion huts."[10]

Murphy's description sharpens our understanding of the marginalized status commonly attributed to people with disabilities. While progress has been made, stigmatizing influences continue to affect our perceptions surrounding disability.[11]

Disability scholars and advocates often criticize Western medicine for its historical view of disability as pathology requiring disease management, and families as unable to cope or to participate effectively in self-care related to the disabling condition.[12] Contemporary family science frameworks and research findings for families with disabled children reflect a changing psycho-socio-cultural context for disability and movement away from a historical emphasis on mourning, stress, and family dysfunction in families with disabled children.[13]

The sociopolitical definition for disability provides a socially constructed, minority-group model. Differences associated with disability are viewed as normative; the problem exists within the environment rather than in the person. Remediation efforts focus on removal of attitudinal, architectural, sensory, and economic barriers. Perceived problems include inadequate support services to overcome these barriers and may include overdependence on professionals.[14] I believe that many health professionals are unaware of these definitional shifts and practice from an illness-based model for disability.

Although the Christian church offers the "language of inclusiveness," Gourgey[15] observes that people within the church, similar to those outside of

10. Robert F. Murphy, *The Body Silent* (New York: Henry Holt, 1990), pp. 106, 122, 135.

11. Robert P. Marinelli and Arthur E. Dell Orto, eds., *The Psychological and Social Impact of Disability,* 4th ed. (New York: Springer, 1999); Mark Nagler, ed., *Perspectives on Disability: Text and Readings on Disability* (Palo Alto, Calif.: Health Markets Research, 1993).

12. Philip M. Ferguson, Alan Gartner, and Dorothy Lipsky, "Research on Families of Children with Disabilities: A Brief Review and Commentary" (Garrison, N.Y.: Hastings Center Project on Genetic Testing and Disability, 1997), pp. 1-18.

13. Mary Frances Hanline, "Transitions and Critical Events in the Family Life Cycle: Implications for Providing Support to Families of Children with Disabilities," *Psychology in the Schools* 28, no. 1 (1991): 53-59.

14. David Pfeiffer, "Overview of the Disability Movement: History, Legislative Record, and Political Implications," *Policy Studies Journal* 21, no. 4 (1993): 724-34.

15. Charles Gourgey, "From Weakness to Strength: A Spiritual Response to Disability," *Journal of Religion in Disability and Rehabilitation* 1, no. 1 (1994): 69-80.

the church, may see people with disabilities as "outsiders" or a "separate and perhaps unreachable group." Despite good intentions, Creamer writes: "The fact of their ignorance does not make the pain they inflict any less."[16] Similar to the public, the church's predominant response to the population is pity, paternalism, or avoidance. Too often, churches may relate to people with disabilities as those who are *different, not the same* as others.

Despite theological and sociocultural obstacles, there are more positive than negative functions of religiousness in families with disabled members. Religious belief systems, apart from formalized religious practice, may promote acceptance and provide a way for families to give meaning to the disability.[17] Contrary to positive findings, however, parents may experience increased stress associated with religion, including perception of religious failure or punishment for wrongdoing. In some cases, parents turn away from religion.[18]

Because we are thinking, feeling, spiritual beings, we seek to understand the reason and purpose for disability. Our questions include the following: "Who am I and what does disability mean for my life?" "Why me? Why now?" "What did I do to deserve this?" "How can a 'good' God allow this?" "Did God cause this?" "Why doesn't God heal me (or my child): Do I lack faith?"

While most religious traditions address suffering, those who seek theological explanations for disability will seldom find a clearly articulated single answer.[19] The problem becomes magnified with lack of clear or adequate teaching from a biblical perspective.[20] In the midst of theological confusion and public attitudes surrounding the meaning of disability, people with dis-

---

16. Deborah Creamer, "Finding God in Our Bodies: Theology from the Perspective of People with Disabilities, Part 1," *Journal of Religion in Disability and Rehabilitation* 2, no. 1 (1995): 28.

17. Tess Bennett, Deborah A. Deluca, and Robin W. Allen, "Religion and Children with Disabilities," *Journal of Religion and Health* 34, no. 4 (1995): 301-12; Michael Wrigley and Mark LaGory, "The Role of Religion and Spirituality in Rehabilitation: A Sociological Perspective," *Journal of Religion in Disability and Rehabilitation* 1, no. 3 (1994): 27-40.

18. Thomas S. Weisner, Laura Beizer, and Lori Stolze, "Religion and Families of Children with Developmental Delays," *American Journal on Mental Retardation* 95, no. 6 (1991): 647-62.

19. George W. Paterson, *Helping Your Handicapped Child* (Minneapolis: Augsburg Publishing House, 1975).

20. Nancy L. Eiesland, *The Disabled God: Toward a Liberatory Theology of Disability* (Nashville: Abingdon Press, 1994); Charles Gourgey, "Enlarge the Site of Your Tent: Making a Place in the Church for People with Disabilities," in *And Show Steadfast Love,* ed. Lewis H. Merrick (Louisville, Ky.: Presbyterian Church, 1993), pp. 29-45.

abilities may internalize negative messages; the outcome is rejection of God and spiritual beliefs that could be helpful.[21]

Applications for Health Care Practice

Establishing Meaning for Disability

People affected by disability and the public need *clearly articulated information from the church to assist them to establish theological meaning for disability*. The participants revealed questions surrounding the judgment of God, adequacy of faith, and miraculous healing. Sources of blame for disability included God, self, family, and society.

Barry speaks from personal experience with physical disabilities, and his perspective as a counselor: "I see a lot of breakup in families because of the child who's disabled. . . . The blame has to be put somewhere. They either put it on each other, or they put it on God." When Theresa's multiply-disabled son was born: "I thought God was punishing me. I couldn't believe it! I really had a rough time. I didn't understand how God could give me a problem like this, when I had so many problems to begin with." Another mother, Joyce, says, "I was led to believe that if you do something wrong, if you sin, then God will slap you down. I could have taken Carl's cerebral palsy from God." Prior to the birth of Beth, Marg and Ted discussed adoption of a "handicapped child; at that time it was the in-thing to do. Society thought I was a hero when I discussed adopting, and blamed me when I had one of my own." Ted, chuckling wryly, says that the decision to have four children rather than two, in addition to the birth of a child with disabilities, made them a "blemish on society."

The participants used their spiritual beliefs to create meaning for disability, in the midst of social stigma and theological confusion. Both adults with disabilities and family members complained about the church's lack of assistance with establishing meaning for disability. Bill, a father who attended mainline Protestant churches and a nondenominational Bible church on a regular basis for more than forty years, expresses his frustration: "If the pulpit never says anything about disabled [persons] then my thought process is that Jesus never addressed the issue." Bill believes that his lack of a biblical foundation for understanding of disability allowed Satan to tempt him years earlier with thoughts that God was punishing him through failure of miraculous

---

21. Gourgey, "From Weakness to Strength."

healing for his daughter, Cathy. He, similar to others, moved away from God as a result. Another parent, Connie, says: "I would have liked to have had somebody tell me, instead of me having to read that my child is the way he is because God did it or allowed it." In the absence of assistance by pastoral leaders, Connie found help through reading a practical Christian text.[22]

Theological confusion surrounding disability continues within and outside of the church. Caregivers who work with disabled persons can encourage their religious institutions to openly address disability and its associated issues of God's judgment, adequacy of faith, miraculous healing, and suffering from a scriptural perspective. This requires that churches evaluate historical positions that have been assumed without careful study of theological issues surrounding disability.

As professionals, however, our interventions must extend beyond efforts to influence religious leaders and institutions. A holistic focus on mind, body, and spirit promotes recognition and achievement of spiritual needs surrounding disability.[23] Our assessments should include key questions and other strategies that invite communication about spiritual needs and concerns. Receptivity to others' spiritual needs requires comfort with our own spirituality. In talking directly with the patient and family about these issues, we should not demand that others accept our views on spirituality. We can collaborate with pastoral staff and qualified counselors as they help individuals and families grapple with spiritual issues surrounding disability. Our resource network should include churches that have demonstrated acceptance and support of people with disabilities and others perceived to be different.

Establishing meaning for disability and reconciliation of blame for a child with disabilities appear essential to family and marital harmony. Early intervention efforts in families affected by disability are typically directed toward mothers; they should include fathers and siblings. Cathy, a young adult with disabilities, suggested that disabled children need opportunities to establish theological meaning for disability apart from their parents. Most participants, however, agreed that it is unlikely that families will ask for this kind of assistance: It has typically not been available and the majority of the participants do not expect the church to minister to them in this way. Both parents and adults with disabilities believe that *churches should initiate* these kinds of

22. James Dobson, *When God Doesn't Make Sense* (Wheaton, Ill.: Tyndale House, 1993).

23. Treloar, "Spiritual Care: Assessment and Intervention," *Journal of Christian Nursing* 16, no. 2 (1999): 15-18.

contacts and discussions. *Open and direct discussion of disability should occur at multiple levels.*

While health professionals who integrate spiritual care into their practice cannot replace members of the clergy, they can collaborate with church leaders to help people ascribe meaning to disability and provide continuing religious support. This requires familiarity with theological explanations for questions surrounding disability. Following his spinal cord injury, Jim found that the counsel of well-meaning Christians was not helpful because it was not biblically based. Jim comments:

> Christians would come in to visit me in the hospital. Most of them would have some sort of answer. They'd say, "I feel this or that about your accident. This is why it happened. God has a reason for these things." *It was not comforting to have somebody saying that God has a reason for this when you're in the middle of it.*
>
> One pastor . . . said, "For every non-Christian who has an injury or an accident of some kind, God puts a Christian through the same sort of ordeal to show the world the difference." I said, "No, it's not. Just stop! That's no help. I know you're trying to help, but that isn't any help at all. The things that might be true, but you don't know are true, let's not waste the time on it. Because you don't know." . . . *Only those things that God said to us in the Bible, those were the only things that were true and helpful and nurturing to me.*

Persons who effectively minister to people affected by disability and their families provide a *spiritually sensitive presence that does not need to offer "answers" to disability.* Counsel given in response to the person/family's request for direction, however, should reflect scriptural truths.

Disability deeply affects the relationships of disabled and nondisabled persons. One young adult described emotional barriers between herself and her mother, emanating from her health problems secondary to spina bifida. Karen comments on perceptual differences between her and her parents:

> Even when I continue to suffer as an adult, it's like they [parents] don't recognize all that I go through emotionally because of my disability. They think that I'm doing real well. I think they're so scarred by what they suffered that they can't look at what I suffered as much as what they suffered.

Jim and his wife, Angela, complained about others' lack of understanding of their situation; at the same time, they recognized that prior to Jim's accident, they did not understand disability. Jim says:

It's real easy to see who's suffered and who hasn't suffered in close friends that I have. I think it's so easy because I was one of those people. I knew two or three quadriplegics, but I had no clue. I didn't know what to say to them, I didn't know how to relate to them. I felt uncomfortable around them. . . . I had no idea what it was like to be disabled.

Both Jim and Angela complained about others' lack of understanding of their experience. Yet Angela found that she, similar to others, was unexplainably stopped from showing compassion to Jim. One day in the hospital his body lay at an angle that resembled the bodies of geriatric patients she had cared for in the past. This revolted her. The literature calls this "aesthetic aversion."[24] Angela's personal response to the physical changes in Jim remains troubling to her, eighteen months after his accident. She says:

> I was totally revolted by the whole thing. I felt so guilty. Talk about having no compassion. . . . I didn't have compassion for Jim. And I still don't to a certain degree. It's like there's a part of my heart that can't come to grips. Something inhibits me from showing compassion to Jim. He wants me to rub his legs. I don't have the compassion to do it. That's terrible. It bothers me greatly. Of course, he can't understand why. Really I don't either.

One of the threads that run through the participants' stories is others' lack of understanding and failure to demonstrate compassion toward them. Too often others responded out of "pity." Yet Angela, strangely enough, experienced the same kinds of reservations in serving Jim that the participants complained about.

Mary commented that she feels lonely when her son Paul is hospitalized, despite the presence of visitors. She, too, remains isolated; people hold themselves back from participating in her pain. Mary says:

> Every time Paul's been in the hospital, that's the most lonesome time with everybody around me. It's like, "What are you all doing? Where is your concern?" It's like they're putting on a facade — we did our thing. We came and visited and said our prayers. But, I could feel the — "Don't let me get too close, for fear I'll hurt."

Both adults with disabilities and family members described a deep pain associated with the experience of disability that others cannot or do not choose to join in. Angela says:

24. Hanoch Livneh, "On the Origins of Negative Attitudes Toward People with Disabilities," *Rehabilitation Literature* 43, no. 11-12 (1982): 338-47.

I began to see so clearly through this whole experience how many people there were, that because they had never experienced suffering, *they didn't know what suffering was, deep suffering of the heart.* . . . *They had to give us answers to make themselves feel better.* . . . It was just upsetting to us at the time.

The participants wanted their needs to be met on practical and spiritual levels that convey understanding of their experience. Despite our status as health professionals, we may not understand the experience of disability; we should not pretend to do otherwise. We must open our senses to the experiences of others. Practical gestures as simple as offering a cup of coffee or a blanket to a family member convey caring in a fast-paced health-care environment. Difference and illness create isolation; opportunities for sharing of feelings associated with these events must be provided. *Deeply listening promotes spiritual well-being.* At the end of his family's interview, Ted said, "I think there's healing just in talking about this today." Professionals who utilize these strategies can improve the way they accompany people with disabilities on their journeys through life.

We must be aware of our attitudes and the way in which we render assistance to others. Cathy, a young adult with disabilities, proposed a theory for people's responses to her, based on her observation as to whether they had achieved meaning for disability. Cathy comments:

A Christian who does not have a conclusion about disability will assist someone who is disabled simply because it's the right thing to do, it's a good deed they're supposed to do. I don't like that. If people really want to help me, then I want their help, but I don't want their pity. . . . A non-Christian who does not have a belief system [about the meaning for disability] will not do it [help me], because they don't want to. They will be up front. I would prefer that, rather than a Christian doing it because they're supposed to.

In Cathy's observations, help rendered from obligation conveys pity, rather than compassion. When we choose to help because it's the right thing to do, rather than because we want to, our actions become uncaring. If we cannot do our work with joy, it may be time to do something else. Ask yourself: *How are you serving others?*

When Jim was hospitalized following his accident, the most helpful health-care professionals asked his opinion; they invited his participation in his care. He contrasted the actions and attitude of a nurse who demonstrated compassion toward him, with those whom he perceived as patronizing. He says:

When she came into the room she treated me as a person, as an adult, as a 29-year-old-male, as a peer. She had to do everything for me. Clean me up, brush, whatever. But that's how she treated me. The other extreme of that are the people who were patronizing to me, who would just as soon give me a pill and put me out as they would go a ways to help me. . . . There were two nurses that I dreaded. For me it was a nightmare to have them come in. Then there are the other people too, who would never leave me alone, who mothered me to death.

The first nurse maintained Jim's worth and value as a peer; his physical limitations were incidental, not primary. The others belittled him: he took on the role of a child, they acted as parents. *Compassion maintains worth of the person; pity offers help while it squashes the recipient's self.*

Support of People Affected by Disability Begins with You

Effective interactions with people affected by disability begin with personal awareness of your thoughts and feelings surrounding disability. Ask yourself: "Do my actions support stigma, isolation, and devaluation of people with disabilities?" "Am I sensitive to cultural differences in response to and support of this population?" Interdisciplinary professionals who are attuned to family stresses and available social support programs provide hope for families mired in the difficulties of their daily lives. Our skills may prepare us to facilitate a community-based small group that promotes networking of families and resources in the community. Private and public social support systems continue to lag far behind needs. We can become involved in social issues and programs that provide services to people affected by disability, furnishing needed leadership and expertise to the community.

Professionals who understand the population's issues and concerns are ably suited to collaborate with people affected by disability, advocate for them, and teach others about this population within our churches. More importantly, we can help empower people affected by disabilities to take an active role in their congregations; to fully participate in the spiritual life of the church.

Chronic sorrow may exist alongside joy for people with disabilities and their families. In my study, adults with disabilities and family members saw their lives as serving a purpose. They chose to live with joy and thankfulness despite difficulties associated with disability. Professionals who assist people affected by disability to achieve spiritual well-being promote health that transcends physical, cognitive, or emotional limitations. Moltmann describes health, as it incorporates spiritual elements: "True health is the strength to live, the strength to suffer, and the strength to die. Health is not a condition of my body; it is the power of my soul to cope with the varying condition of that body."[25]

What is your view of health for people with disabilities? When we insist on seeing things from our perspective, we influence potential outcomes. Disability changes the way in which persons with disabilities accomplish tasks and meet needs. The public may view disability as burdensome, and the actions of parents of disabled children and persons with disabilities as heroic. The data, however, suggest that people who effectively adapt to disability choose to view difficulties associated with disability differently from those who do not share their experience.

Cathy, who uses a power wheelchair and relies on assistance by others for activities of daily living, reframes what appear to be overwhelming and repeated struggles or burdens as "challenges." Life becomes an "obstacle course with a way to get to the other end. Just have to do it a bit differently — not the conventional means. I have speed bumps, doors, and windows, all those different types of metaphors."

Accommodation to life's challenges associated with disability may occur differently from our view of the ideal situation. We cannot assume that our perspectives for health and quality of life represent those of people affected by disability. Professionals should promote self-care and participation in personal health care: We must plan *with*, rather than *for*, the person and family. This requires open communication, unrestrained by power and position differences.

Consistent with the contemporary sociopolitical model for disability, we must attempt to alleviate environmental limitations that impair a disabled person's ability to live life to the same extent as a nondisabled person. To this end, we need to cultivate the ability to see through the eyes of someone affected by disability. An interdisciplinary team perspective that places the person and the family at its head, and that extends into the community, is needed. People with disabilities may be different, but *they are created in the image of God*, the same as people unaffected by disability.

Since love for God and love for another (Matt. 22:37-40) lie at the heart of a biblical ethical perspective for the church's relationship with people affected by disability, Christians ought to ask: *What does it mean to live as the body of Christ?* How does this direct our lives as disabled and nondisabled

---

25. Jürgen Moltmann, "The Liberation and Acceptance of the Handicapped," in *The Power of the Powerless* (San Francisco: Harper and Row, 1983), p. 142.

persons in Christian community? This central principle must guide the practice of health professionals and leaders of our churches as we join with people affected by disability in serving one another.

PART V

THE CHURCH

The Church and the
Cultural Imperative

C. Ben Mitchell, Ph.D.

When Richard Weaver published his 1948 classic volume, *Ideas Have Conse-quences* (Chicago: University of Chicago Press), he could not have imagined the mammoth consequences the *idea of bioethics* would have. In its contem-porary incarnation, the idea of bioethics had its genesis in two phenomena: (1) the abuse of human subjects in research and (2) flexible plastic tubing. The first of those phenomena is probably self-explanatory and the second will become obvious with just a moment of reflection. Were it not for flexible plastic tubing, we could not keep patients alive on ventilators and IVs. With-out flexible plastic tubing, there would be very few end-of-life decisions to make. Without flexible plastic tubing, kidney dialysis would not be feasible. Without flexible plastic tubing, certain diagnostic procedures would be im-possible. Without flexible plastic tubing, many patients would die of uremic poisoning, since catheters could not be placed. One seemingly inauspicious technology turned the world of medicine upside down and launched an idea with very auspicious consequences.

Similarly, the idea of the church has consequences. The affirmation of the Apostles' Creed, "I believe in . . . the holy catholic church, the communion of the saints . . . ," is an idea with momentous consequences. But the *communio sanctorum* was not a self-originating idea dreamed up in the smoke-filled back rooms of a hovel in Jerusalem. Our confession is that the idea of the church originated in the mind of God. What might be thought to be a very inauspicious idea, with very meager beginnings, has had very auspi-cious consequences.

Unlike many other institutions, God's idea of the church includes cultural engagement. In fact, there is a divine mandate for churchly engagement with the *kosmos*.[1] We are called to be salt and light in the *kosmos* (Matt. 5:13-16). Neither separatist nonengagement nor total cultural preoccupation are options for the church facing the twenty-first century. The necessity of churchly involvement in the culture has never been greater and cutting-edge bioethical and public policy issues should be arenas of crucial engagement for the church.

What do we mean by "engagement"? And how do we "engage" the culture? What is the role of the church in this "engagement"? These are the questions I will address. One brief aside: since my assignment is to deal with the topic of making a difference through the church, I will use churchly language to talk about the role of the church. That is to say, I am couching my argument very self-consciously in theological language, using a theological paradigm consistent with the Christian tradition.

Because I believe that the churchly paradigm given to us in Scripture at one and the same time gives us both a definition and example of what churchly engagement with the *kosmos* looks like, I want to use that theological paradigm as a way of getting at our subject. Therefore, I want to examine our subject — making a difference through the church — under the rubric of three imperatives that belong to the church: the prophetic imperative, the Samaritan imperative, and the conservative imperative.

The Prophetic Imperative — Jeremiah 1:1-10

The words of Jeremiah the son of Hilkiah, of the priests who were in Anathoth in the land of Benjamin, to whom the word of the Lord came in the days of Josiah the son of Amon, king of Judah, in the thirteenth year of his reign. It came also in the days of Jehoiakim the son of Josiah, king of Judah, until the end of the eleventh year of Zedekiah the son of Josiah, king of Judah, until the carrying away of Jerusalem captive in the fifth month.

The word of the Lord came to me saying, "Before I formed you in the womb I knew you; Before you were born I sanctified you; I ordained you a prophet to the nations." Then said I: Ah, Lord God! Behold, I cannot speak, for I am a youth." But the Lord said to me: "Do not say, 'I am a youth,' For you shall go to all to whom I send you, And whatever I command you, you shall speak. Do not be afraid of their faces, For I am with you to deliver

---

1. For an exposition of the importance of *kosmos* for bioethics, see the chapter in this volume by John F. Kilner, "A Biblical Mandate for Cultural Engagement."

you," says the Lord. Then the Lord put forth His hand and touched my mouth, and the Lord said to me: "Behold, I have put My words in your mouth. See, I have this day set you over the nations and over the kingdoms, To root out and pull down, To destroy and throw down, To build and to plant."

The Old Testament uses three words to designate a prophet, *nabhi*, *ro'eh*, and *chozeh*. *Nabhi*, the most common word for prophet, is a word that carries the idea of "bubbling up." The prophet spoke as the word of God bubbled up, like an artesian spring, within his mind and heart. When the word "prophet" is used in the Greek New Testament, it translates a word that means "to speak forth" *(prophemi)*. According to Peter, ". . . no prophecy of scripture is of any private interpretation, for prophecy never came by the will of man, but holy men of God spoke as they were moved by the Holy Spirit" (2 Peter 1:20). Thus, the prophet had the following traits:

- uncompromisingly committed to God's word;
- conscious of a divine call to speak that word;
- aware of and humbled by the privilege of access to the counsel of God;
- a person of decided action;
- conscious of divine authority;
- in communion with God;
- an individual of personal holiness;
- addresses specific evils; and
- only lastly, an agent to reveal the future.

Just as God called individuals to the prophetic office in the Old Testament, and just as our Lord Jesus functioned in his prophetic office — speaking the word of truth — so the church is to exercise her prophetic voice to "speak forth the word of the Lord." As anyone knows who reads the prophets, the words of the prophets were meant primarily as a communication from God to his people. The prophets declared the word of the Lord to the people of the Lord.

The first thing we must do to make a difference through the church is to speak the word of the Lord to the church. That is to say, our first responsibility is an educational responsibility — speaking forth the word of the Lord and calling the church to repentance and obedience.

In his thought-provoking and convicting volume, *The Christian Mind: How Should a Christian Think?* Harry Blamires observed in 1963: "there is no longer a Christian mind." Thirty-six years later, it's not clear to me that the church is any closer to having a Christian mind than we were when Blamires penned those haunting words. This unfortunate situation exists despite the fact that we are commanded in Scripture: "Do not be conformed to this world, but be transformed by the renewing of your mind, that you may prove what is the good and acceptable and perfect will of God" (Rom. 12:2). The church has invested hundreds of billions of dollars in Christian schools of higher education over the centuries as a response to this exhortation.

I am convinced that the reason we are so ineffectual in developing a Christian mind is because the church (or, perhaps more importantly, the churches) is not committed to doing so. Either we are distracted by a noble but misdirected pietism; or we are being anesthetized by mind-numbing pabulum; or we are, as theologian Alister McGrath puts it, "wandering aimlessly from one 'meaningful' issue to another in a desperate search for relevance in the eyes of the world."[2] *If we do not cultivate Christian worldview thinking we cannot engage the culture, make a difference, nor properly worship God with all of our mind.* Dorothy L. Sayers develops this line of thought in the following manner:

> The one thing I am here to say to you is this: that it is worse than useless for Christians to talk about the importance of Christian morality, unless they are prepared to take their stand upon the fundamentals of Christian theology. It is a lie to say that dogma does not matter; it matters enormously. It is fatal to let people suppose that Christianity is only a mode of feeling; it is virtually necessary to insist that it is first and foremost a rational explanation of the universe. It is hopeless to offer Christianity as a vaguely idealistic aspiration of a simple and consoling kind; it is, on the contrary, a hard, tough, exacting and complex doctrine, steeped in a drastic and uncompromising realism.[3]

Christian morality is dependent on Christian doctrine. Christian doctrine is dependent on scriptural revelation. Christian minds are dependent on scriptural understanding.

How can the church make a difference without having a Christian mind? How will we call the church to the cultivation of the Christian mind? How will we address the issues before us faithfully if we do not cultivate Christian worldview thinking? Let me at least suggest that we need curricular help along these lines. The church needs serious educational curricula in

---

2. Alister E. McGrath, "Doctrine and Ethics," in *Readings in Christian Ethics,* ed. David K. Clark and Robert V. Rakestraw, vol. 1 (Grand Rapids: Baker Books, 1994), p. 89.
3. McGrath, "Doctrine and Ethics," p. 85.

bioethics. If, as some futurists are suggesting, the twenty-first century will be the biotech century, how can we have any hope at all of interpreting, addressing, and engaging these issues unless the church cultivates a Christian mind on these matters? How can local churches, members of the body of Christ, cultivate a Christian mind on these matters without scientifically accurate and biblically faithful educational resources?

The intellectual and professional leaders of the church must take up the prophetic mantle and call the church to obedience in this area. If they will not, who will? If they do not do it now, when? Until the church develops an informed mind on the bioethical agenda of the culture, our prophetic ministry to the *kosmos* will be impotent at best and harmful at worst. Another important component of the prophetic imperative is speaking to the world. But we cannot speak effectively to the world, while our own house is so disorderly.

The Samaritan Imperative — Luke 10:30-37

A certain man went down from Jerusalem to Jericho, and fell among thieves, who stripped him of his clothing, wounded him, and departed, leaving him half dead. Now by chance a certain priest came down that road. And when he saw him, he passed by on the other side. Likewise a Levite, when he arrived at the place, came and looked, and passed by on the other side. But a certain Samaritan, as he journeyed, came where he was. And when he saw him, he had compassion. So he went to him and bandaged his wounds, pouring on oil and wine; and he set him on his own animal, brought him to an inn, and took care of him. On the next day, when he departed, he took out two denarii, gave them to the innkeeper, and said to him, "Take care of him; and whatever more you spend, when I come again, I will repay you." So which of these three do you think was neighbor to him who fell among the thieves? And [the man] said, "He who showed mercy on him." Then Jesus said to him, "Go and do likewise."

Note the imperative, *"Go and do likewise"* (v. 37). We must face the fact that some Christians are just not going to be deep thinkers. In fact, some are easily bored exercising their minds. The prophetic ministry may not be for all Christians. Some of our brothers and sisters just want something they can do. Thus, another important way to engage the *kosmos* is through hands-on ministry to suffering people. Samaritan ministry is not optional for Christians, it is an imperative.

Let me provide one example of a church that is living out the Samaritan imperative. First Baptist Church of Leesburg, Florida, has a phenomenal ministry. Pastor Charles Rosell says that along with the regular teaching and preaching ministry of the church, First Baptist Leesburg operates on its campus:

- a rescue mission that serves a hundred persons;
- a women's shelter for twenty women and children;
- an emergency children's home that has housed 1,200 children this year;
- a teen home for twenty teens at a time;
- a pregnancy care center that serves about 125 women per month;
- a Rapha counseling ministry;
- a before- and after-school care ministry;
- a day-care center for children; and
- a furniture barn and food pantry of 5,000-square feet.

The pastor estimates that last year the church provided $1,800 per day to ministry and gave $1,000 per day to missions. Nearly all of these ministries are staffed by volunteers.

In addition, First Baptist Church is building a medical center for the uninsured in conjunction with a local hospital. The hospital is donating over $650,000. Twenty doctors and nurses have volunteered their services. At the end of ten years the church will own the center completely. The hospital agreed to the following conditions:

1. The church will have total control of the ministry.
2. The church will present the gospel of Christ to everyone who comes to the center.
3. Abortion is not negotiable.
4. No contraceptives will be distributed to minors.

All of this is in a town of 15,000, in a county of approximately 50,000. We are not talking about a metropolis. Why do other churches not undertake these kinds of ministries? Certainly because they have not cultivated a Christian mind. Clearly because they have not caught the Samaritan imperative.

The need for Samaritan care is not lessening in our culture, but becoming greater. If our world continues to embrace the culture of death and increasingly supports legalized assisted dying, churches will need to establish crisis dying centers just like they had to build crisis pregnancy centers. Just as many pregnant women need places of refuge where they can escape the pressure to abort their unborn babies, so dying patients will need communities of care where they can die without pressure to end their lives prematurely. Church-operated hospice and, perhaps a return to church-based charitable hospitals, has to be a part of our Samaritan strategy.

Some ethicists and policymakers may be able to mount a strong and persuasive argument against universal health-care insurance, but they cannot excise the Samaritan imperative from Scripture. Neighborly love requires that we strategize ways of ministering to those who are not insured.

The Conservative Imperative — 2 Timothy 1:8-14

Therefore do not be ashamed of the testimony of our Lord, nor of me His prisoner, but share with me in the sufferings for the gospel according to the power of God, who has saved us and called us with a holy calling, not according to our works, but according to His own purpose and grace which was given to us in Christ Jesus before the world began, but has now been revealed by the appearing of your Savior Jesus Christ, who has abolished death and brought life and immortality to light through the gospel, to which I was appointed a preacher, an apostle, and a teacher of the Gentiles. For this reason also I suffer these things; nevertheless I am not ashamed, for I know whom I have believed and am persuaded that He is able to keep what I have committed to Him until that Day.

Hold fast the pattern of sound words which you have heard from me, in faith and love which are in Christ Jesus. That good thing which was committed to you, keep by the Holy Spirit who dwells in us.

The imprisoned apostle writes to the young minister, Timothy, and by extension to the church, to "hold fast the pattern of sound words" which he had heard from Paul. I take that to mean, among other things, that the church is to be a conservator of the truth, holding fast the tradition, maintaining the body of doctrine committed to the church.

"Holding fast the pattern of sound words" entails, in my view, not capitulating to the language of secular bioethics, even in the arena of public policy. For instance, the first principle of contemporary secular bioethics is autonomy. But autonomy is not a biblical notion; at least not the way it is formulated by most people. *Auto-nomos* (self-law) is a decidedly anti-Christian idea. In fact, we could argue that at the heart of the sinful human condition is the desire for *auto-nomos*. The false autonomy so characteristic of our culture and so embedded in contemporary bioethics is not an idea, or even a word, we ought to proliferate.

Instead, a Christian worldview replaces self-determination with responsibility. "You are not your own, you've been bought with a price. Therefore, glorify God in your body and in your spirit which are God's" (1 Cor. 6:19b, 20), we are told. Our lives are not our own. We cannot create them by our will and we may not end them by our will. The church must not slowly give away the notion of responsibility in favor of more high-sounding principles like autonomy, or even rights. The unborn may have a "right to life," but an unborn child cannot act on that right. We have a moral responsibility not to kill the unborn or use them in experimentation. Terminally ill patients may have a right to life, but they are hardly able to defend that right in the end-stages of lung cancer. We have a moral responsibility to care for the dying. I fear that "rights" language often removes the onus of responsibility from those to whom it properly belongs. The church must mind her language, holding fast the pattern of sound words as a conservator of the truth.

Another example: We have been told that in order to engage the culture we have to sanitize our language of all religious concepts. Ronald Dworkin says, for instance, that "Political decisions must be, so far as is possible, independent of any particular conception of the good life, or what gives value to life." This statement has a ring of neutrality about it. Policy matters are supposed to be neutral with respect to "any particular conception of the good life." *But, isn't that very statement a conception of the good life?* The idea that policy must be neutral is a myth. There can be no such thing as neutral conception of the good life.[4]

This is not to say that we have to cite chapter and verse for every policy recommendation. All that is being said here is that public policies should be compatible with traditional religious principles which have withstood the test of time. Since ideas have consequences, we must not sacrifice that which we hold sacred on the altar of so-called public discourse.

I spend a fair amount of time in a variety of dialogues on religion and bioethics. These dialogues usually include twenty or thirty people sitting around a table, each supposedly representing a different theological or cultural tradition, all trying to speak the moral Esperanto of secular bioethics. It is tempting to emulate one's colleagues in these dialogues and try to cast one's convictions in secular terms. Instead, we are called to translate our conception of the good into images that can be grasped by our culture. We are not

---

4. For a book-length debate on this topic by two Christian thinkers, see Robert Audi and Nicholas Wolterstorff, *Religion in the Public Square: The Place of Religious Convictions in Political Debate* (Lanham, Md.: Rowman and Littlefield, 1997). My own view is closer to Wolterstorff than Audi.

permitted to capitulate our conception of the good for the sake of sounding respectable and cordial. The siren song of secularism is difficult to resist.

We must maintain our confessional fidelity if we are to maintain our integrity. If the church gives up that which we distinctively have to offer, namely, "a particular conception of the good life," she has nothing to offer. Hold fast the pattern of sound words!

*　　*　　*

What happens if we don't prevail? How long does the church "hold fast"? How long does she engage? Frankly, until our Lord's return. *We will make a difference* if we obey the prophetic imperative, calling the church back to repentance and calling her to worship God with the mind, developing a Christian worldview perspective on the matters before us. *We will make a difference* if we obey the Samaritan imperative, engaging the culture in transformative ministry. And *we will make a difference* by remaining faithful to the faith once for all delivered to the saints, even in the face of transience of the postmodern ethos.

How do we measure our success? Some have observed that during the so-called Dark Ages of the church, those who were responsible for the survival of the Christian faith were those quiet, unassuming monks who faithfully, day after day, copied and preserved the Scriptures. Those monks maintained the repository of truth for a future generation. Similarly, we ought to measure our success not by our numbers, but by our fidelity to truth.

Frankly, we may not see the day when human life is protected from conception to natural death. We may not see the day when medicine is restored to its covenantal character. We may not see the day when ethically responsible research means that human embryos will not have to be killed. We may not see the day when assisted suicide is outlawed in all fifty states again.

But our grandchildren, or their children's children, may ask one day, "did anyone protest the spirit of the age? Did anyone offer a better way? Did anyone try to protect the dignity of human persons?" And, perhaps, they'll find the proceeding of this conference or uncover the written works of many faithful Christian scholars and say, "yes, someone did point us to a better way. Our way is a dismal failure. Let us try what they said. Perhaps that will make a difference!"

Biblical Context for
the Church's Bioethics

R. Geoffrey Brown, Ph.D.

America's Modern Voice

The elemental moral dissonance in America's modern cultural voice presents a huge challenge to enacting biblical truth in bioethics. Thomas C. Oden, professor of theology at Drew University, has noted that a certain "mod rot" is advancing on contemporary American culture.[1] It's moving in political, economic, and ecclesiastical arenas. The nagging question for the church is, just how strongly has the culture's at-times miasmic voice impacted Christians who themselves are called to transform decaying cultural voices with a bioethical biblical freshness?

In order to counteract the sometimes insidious strength of the culture, Christians desiring to make a cultural difference in doing bioethics will want to have a biblically balanced threefold presuppositional approach. Christians will want to have a threefold confidence born out of an intentional identity, which has arisen through a triad of redemptive supernaturalism, rather than an identity rising from undiscerned processes of acculturation and socialization.

This threefold presuppositional approach may be stated as follows. It's

---

1. Thomas Oden, *Two Worlds: Notes on the Death of Modernity in America and Russia* (Downers Grove, Ill.: InterVarsity Press, 1992), p. 17. Oden notes that a "mod rot" has infected political and economic arenas in both Russia and the USA. For further elucidation on what I have called here "the cultural voice," see chapter 2, "Postmodern Consciousness," pp. 31-47.

based upon the apostle Paul's writings as the word of God. But since the written word of God is unified by divine plenary verbal inspiration, the three ethically inextricable premises here would find validation essentially throughout the entirety of holy Scripture. They are as follow:

- First, to make a difference in bioethics, Christians must act with confident expectation rising out of their intentional identity as *new creation;*
- Second, to make a difference in bioethics, Christians must engender confident encouragement sustained by their intentional identity with the *cross of Christ;* and
- Third, to make a difference in bioethics, Christians must persist with confident endurance provoked by their intentional primary identity first as a member of *community,* rather than first as an individual in America, or perhaps another country of Western civilization.

New Creation, Cross, and Community[2]

These three may be called action frames from which the church acts to make a difference. It's from this biblical triad that Christians are divinely authorized to enter the bioethical culture acting with confident expectation, confident encouragement, and confident endurance — for such is the promise of future grace given in Jesus Christ the Lord to be sufficiently with them in all their focused efforts to glorify God (2 Cor. 12:9).[3]

Interestingly though, just because these three action frames are biblical, in today's society, they are instantly countercultural. As such they are constantly challenged by the prevailing albeit decaying tones of the American modern and postmodern cultural voice. Many sly accents have combined over time and have become interdependently linked to make our culture's voice so influential it's even ecclesiastically invasive.

---

2. I am indebted to Dr. Richard B. Hays for this threefold delineation. See Richard B. Hays, *The Moral Vision of the New Testament: A Contemporary Introduction to New Testament Ethics* (San Francisco: HarperCollins Publishers, 1996), pp. 19-36.

3. This brief paper cannot do justice, but should, to the overriding and supreme motivation for all ethical endeavors and behavior: God's passion for his own glory and our consequent alignment of heart, soul, mind, and strength to value what God himself values, and to enact every ethical effort with our own responsive pursuit of his greater glory. See John Piper, *God's Passion for His Glory: Living the Vision of Jonathan Edwards (With the Complete Text of "The End for Which God Created the World")* (Wheaton, Ill.: Crossway Books, 1998), especially part 2, pp. 117-253.

Cultural Cacophony

Briefly, what are some of these accents and what challenging questions may be summarily posed against them?

One favored cultural accent can be elicited from the slogan, "Have it your way."[4] This patented phrase, seemingly innocent enough in the lunch line, nevertheless captures the prevailing cultural wind of entitlement which has moved people all the way from the mere freedom to make up their own hamburgers to the extent of free choice for euthanasia. Euthanasia, after all, is simply the right to "have it your way" in both life *and* death.

Both churched and unchurched alike are laws to ourselves; this is a dominant personal motif of the modern and postmodern mind. What is this really, however, except the looming cultural icon of autonomous individualism erected tall and visible, shadowing city and ecclesiastical skylines, as well as secular and sacred bioethical deliberations?

Can anything stand against such an attractive yet morally deceptive edifice? Yes, the first bioethical action frame of new creation challenges autonomous individualism with biblical truth indicating that we are not laws to ourselves.

Rather we are a new creation in Christ to be defined by him and his ways, not our own, not our culture's.

A second postmodern accent says, "You only go 'round once, so go for the gusto." This brewery boast moves people all the way from a draft beer in their TGIF hands to the unrestrained entitled pursuit of pleasure all their days. This is nothing less than the encapsulation of narcissistic hedonism: Get all you can for yourself while the getting is good, for after all, you're number one — with complete rights to your own body regarding, for instance, abortion, euthanasia, and cloning.

So what does the church say to this? The bioethical action frame, the cross, runs head on into this by encouraging Christians to count the cost of suffering for the sake of biblical truth coming to bear on bioethical issues. Sacrifice rather than self-fulfillment becomes dominant in the bioethics of ministry. Christians understand themselves as everything *but* number one, although they are profoundly aware that all humanity bears the highest dignity creaturely possible in being made in the image of God.

---

4. Admittedly, certain liberties are about to be taken here and in the paragraphs that follow by infusing via intuitive associations the entirety of a cultural mindset into a hamburger slogan, as well as other catch phrases. The justification for doing this lies in the area of their pedagogical recall as slogans and the hope that difficult abstract concepts will be better understood by connection with them.

A third insidious cultural accent says, "What you see is what you get." This so-called "reality-check" anchor moves the cultural mindset from a mere t-shirt motto all the way to being sunk in the muck of a closed system of fixed inviolable natural laws excluding thereby any comforting concept of a sovereign directing supernatural hand of God. What is this but a catch phrase for reductive naturalism? Its other patented phrase is, "Knock on wood," because that's all there is. Is it any wonder that Dr. Peter Singer, influenced by and moving within this secular context, would define human personhood according to cognitive categories stating that IQ is the determinative standard for valid or invalid human life?[5]

But again, the action frame of new creation says there's much, much more. It says that Christians are caught in the juncture of the already and not yet, the juncture where the promised second coming of Christ is received in down payment by the Holy Spirit within, while Christians still endure the fallenness and brokenness of this age to which they minister Christ's truth. They do so with confident expectation of the constancy of divine providence leading linearly onward to his unstoppable return. The new *kosmos,* though not climactic nor consummate, nevertheless, has already begun. What you see is *not* what you get. It is but a smidgen of what is really out there.

"You say to-may-to and I say to-mah-to; you say po-tay-to and I say po-tah-to — so let's call the whole thing off." This ditty of decaying modernity eventually washes people all the way down the hill into the turbid moral stream of pluralistic relativism. Pluralistic relativism would deny there ever was one sure way of pronouncing words, let alone any way of ever finding moral truth — which as the "X-Files" tells us is out there, but since the FBI's finest, Fox Mulder and Dana Scully, can't find it, neither can you. Implicitly, the cultural message is, "Don't even expect to; all is relative anyway." Certainly, no standards for human cloning or abortion could possibly exist for restricting everyone, although for some they might be relatively relevant. What is definitely unacceptable, however, is the imposition of those personally perceived relevancies on anyone else.

Is it any wonder, then, that in a societal context of a truth-free, value-relative and value neutral, egoistic-pursuing, and anti-theistic culture, the inevitable outcome would be the grotesque overweight Jabba the Hut of them all? It may be called eclectic "tolerationism." Its intimidating antinomian motto is, "Who are you to judge me or anyone else, for that matter?"

5. Peter Singer, "Sanctity of Life or Quality of Life?" *Pediatrics,* July 1983, pp. 128-29.

All Christians adhering to the objectivity of truth know that the only heresy in an American culture holding tolerance as the *summum bonum* or highest ethical value, is if one has standards of truth that infuse love with a discernment declaring right from wrong, acceptable from unacceptable, or in a currently anathematized phrase, *intolerable from tolerable.*

On the other hand, Christians themselves also know that a true system of tolerance inherently consistent with its own standards would of necessity have to "tolerate" positions advocating intolerance, but then who ever said the cultural voice sings on pitch?[6]

Against all this, however, is the third action frame of community. The church as community is to make a difference by intentionally shaping affirmations of limitations, by clearly declaring the intolerable, the bioethically sinful. The community of Christians are the ones divinely authorized to say, "Enough is enough." The community of faith is to say this, for instance, against the genetic juncture of the human species with plant or animal to create the specialized functional chimera.[7]

Ecclesiastical Impact

Unfortunately, however, as intimated above, the persuasive power and nuanced bluntness of these modern accents have not gone unheard in the church.[8] The *Zeitgeist* or spirit of the times is so prevalent and pervasive that its voice of radical freedom getting louder and louder has dinned many Christians' ears to God's own voice of radically defining ethical truth.[9]

6. Francis Schaeffer, *The God Who Is There* (Downers Grove, Ill.: InterVarsity Press, 1979). Dr. Schaeffer shows the inherent inconsistencies within moral relativism, in that people never hold such a position when their own moral values are violated by someone intruding against them. When this happens, Dr. Schaeffer observes, the whole system breaks down, and suddenly standards of absolute behavior qualifications come into play.

7. See R. Geoffrey Brown, "Clones, Chimeras and the Image of God: Lessons from Barthian Bioethics," in *Bioethics and the Future of Medicine: A Christian Appraisal,* ed. John F. Kilner, Nigel M. de S. Cameron, and David L. Schiedermayer (Grand Rapids: Eerdmans, 1995), pp. 238-49.

8. Schaeffer, *The Great Evangelical Disaster* (Westchester, Ill.: Crossway Books, 1984), pp. 43-65, 141-48.

9. John Calvin, *Institutes of the Christian Religion* (Philadelphia: Presbyterian Board of Christian Education, Seventh American Edition), book II, chap. 7, pp. 376-95. Here Calvin sets forth the three uses of God's law with the first being that of a mirror into which the Christian looks. The Christian sees the character of God and his revealed truth and so realizes his or her own needful levels of sanctification by the grace of that law of God.

Over the course of twenty-five years of ordained ministry, I've seen an increasing sense of egregious parishioner entitlement born out of accommodation to modern and postmodern cultural values coupled simultaneously with widespread biblical ignorance.

Christians don't know what God wants anymore, because they don't read what he says anymore. Yet at the same time, they hear constantly what the culture blares incessantly, thereby becoming incorrectly data-based and improperly defined in Christian bioethical approaches.

From a pastor's perspective, it really is time God's church took the following statement from Ecclesiastes both seriously and joyously[10] in a context passionately intellectually desirous of reformation and renewal. Because for the Christian, rather than the *Zeitgeist* being radical freedom, the *Zeitgeist* must be the *Heilige Geist* whom we know to be *die Geist der Wahrheit* (the Spirit of Truth) — in a context of radical love.

Just so, Ecclesiastes 12:13: "Now [that] all has been heard; here is the conclusion of the matter: Fear God and keep his commandments, for this is the whole duty of man."

Without wanting to do any injustice to the singular focus of this text on the life-defining authority of God's Word, nevertheless perhaps it's permissible here creatively to adapt it to say, "Now that all has been heard, here is the conclusion of the matter: Fear God and employ his three undergirding bioethical action frames for making a difference in the church and culture: *new creation, cross, and community*."

These three admittedly are ethically broad: they inform, guide, motivate, authenticate, and life-affirm the impact the church should have in employing particular strategies when particular cultural bioethical challenges arise. These three are the central interlocking frames that surround, undergird, and become the superstructures for holding forth the church's particular bioethical canvases upon which are painted detailed Christian positions for prophetic cultural influence on the specifics. In other words, human stem

---

10. John Piper, *Desiring God: Meditations of a Christian Hedonist* (Sisters, Ore.: Multnomah Books, 1986, 1996). Dr. Piper sets forth the case that God is most glorified in us when we are most delighted and satisfied in him. Hence, it is one thing to obey God out of mere duty. But it is a much higher God-glorifying activity to obey God out of delight in the beauty and majesty of his person as revealed in his holy Word. Dr. Piper uses the illustration that for a man to give flowers to his wife on the wedding anniversary out of mere duty does not duly honor the wife. To give the flowers instead out of sheer delight and joy does rightly honor the wife and the marriage. Just so, in our obedience to God, we are to seek him out of the delight of our souls in who he is and how we love him.

cell research, mapping the humane genome, cloning, euthanasia — all the bioethical issues "for a brave new world."[11]

New Creation

The first of these three bioethical interlocking action frames is simply, new creation. It brings the church confident expectation to make a difference. It's expressed explicitly in 2 Corinthians 5:14-18 (NIV):

> For Christ's love compels us, because we are convinced that one died for all, and therefore all died. And he died for all, that those who live should no longer live for themselves but for him who died for them and was raised again. So from now on we regard no one from a worldly point of view. Though we once regarded Christ in this way, we do so no longer. Therefore, if anyone is in Christ, he is a new creation; the old has gone, the new has come! All this is from God, who reconciled us to himself through Christ and gave us the ministry of reconciliation.

"The old has gone, the new has come" (2 Cor. 5:17b).

If the church is to find its bioethical identity it must do so by confidently locating it within the cosmic drama of God's ushering in of the new age signaled in the death and resurrection of Jesus Christ the Lord. The fifth chapter of 2 Corinthians expresses the fervent prophetic hope for the renewal of the world by God's "new creatures in Christ," his ambassadors, who now carry the ministry of reconciliation.

From the ecclesiastical perspective, this is anything but bioethical passivity, anything but sitting idly by while the medium proclaims the message that postmodern eclectic tolerationism must be tolerated and moral relativism must be hailed in its denial of any truth standards for proper value judgments. Hence, cultural bioethical standards are set by everything but divine revelation. It is a move from theocentricity to egocentricity, and it is our culture.

In contradistinction, however, the very identity of the church is ordained by God to be unabashedly a shaper of people's lives. The community of faith is *supposed to* form people's bioethical perspectives — directly and indirectly. Moreover, when the action frame of new creation is scrutinized it may be seen to give the following important primary motivational quality to

11. John S. Feinberg and Paul D. Feinberg, *Ethics for a Brave New World* (Wheaton, Ill.: Crossway Books, 1993).

Christian bioethics: *confident realistic expectation through the intentionality of new creation identity.*

Intentional Identity

By intentionality is meant Christians' necessary conscious and conscientious biblical self-awareness of already being part of the age to come as the church addresses bioethical issues. Intentionality here means tendentiously and consistently living this out with an intellectual and passionate focus. If Christians stood on their own with mere human resources, they should have no confident expectation of an impact. But in that they are standing at the juncture of a new age, and have tasted its first fruits of redemption and new life in Christ, and are filled with the Holy Spirit, this fuses the church with focused energy and expectation for the cultural engagement.

For the Lord Jesus Christ himself has already ushered Christians into the beginnings of an age yet to be fully realized when he returns. Christians already taste of that age now in salvation, in renewal, in the presence of the Holy Spirit within, in the means of grace as provided for the family of God in the sacraments and in the biblical disciplines of spirituality. Those who believe in Christ are at a cosmic juncture; or, as theologians are fond of saying, they are at the juncture of the already and not yet. Already Christ has come into their lives. They are hidden in God in Christ, already raised up with him and seated at the right hand of the Father. Christ has ushered in a new creation. Christians have become part of this new creation through union of redemption in him. And yet they still wait for all to be fulfilled at his glorious return.

Confident Expectation

How then shall Christians live in the meanwhile of the juncture of the already and the not yet?

The inevitable concomitant to such "new creation" reality is winsomely with confident expectation declaring — lipstyle and lifestyle — the reality of God's truth and love to the surrounding culture, into its morass of confused, often contradictory, ethical options. As already noted, these culturally conflicting options are prompted by the strange admixture of (1) autonomous individualism; (2) narcissistic hedonism; (3) reductive naturalism; (4) pluralistic relativism; and (5) eclectic tolerationism, among others. These are like bumper cars gone wild in the amusement park, sometimes colliding, at other times rolling along side by side.

Therefore, just how action-oriented and intentional should Christians be as God's "new creation"? How pressing is the biblical mandate at this time?

An illustration may be helpful here. Christians are, for example, to be as action-oriented intentional about bringing new creation identity to bear with confident expectation on bioethical decisions as was Women's World Cup Soccer goalie Briana Scurry. On Saturday, July 10, 1999, while the nation watched, Scurry at game's end in the decisive shoot-out soared to deflect China's third penalty shot, setting up the final victory of America to win the Cup. Scurry stepped aggressively forward on China's third shot, guessed left and threw herself in that direction where she met Liu Ying's kick. "I just went totally on instinct," Scurry said. "I knew if I could get one, it would be O.K."[12]

Christians neither guess nor go totally on instinct, although they do have an internal witness of the Holy Spirit within to the authenticity of the Bible as God's written Word and the promise of the sufficiency of future grace that says deeply within, "It will be O.K." Hence, there is a confident expectation derivative from the biblical position of new creation in Christ and the inescapable reality of that fact. That Christians are new creations in Christ, and part of the collective new creation in Christ — this is the God-given warrant for bioethical action to be seen as bioethical obedience to God who has called them into the tension of an existence of the already and not yet. Dr. Richard B. Hays, professor of New Testament at Duke University Divinity School, notes:

> According to Paul, the death and resurrection of Jesus was an apocalyptic event that signaled the end of the old age and portended the beginning of the new. Paul's moral vision is intelligible only when his apocalyptic perspective is kept clearly in mind: the church is to find its identity and vocation by recognizing its role within the cosmic drama of God's reconciliation of the world to himself.[13]

There is also a realism to this confident expectation. This two-age terminology admits to the ongoing existence currently of evil and depredation, but also of the foretaste of the glorious new heaven and new earth yet to come. Hence, Paul describes Christians as those "on whom the ends of the ages have met" (1 Cor. 10:11).

12. Bill Saporito, "What a Kick! What a Team!" *Time* 154, no. 3 (19 July 1999): 58-67.

13. Richard B. Hays, *The Moral Vision of the New Testament: A Contemporary Introduction to New Testament Ethics* (San Francisco: HarperCollins Publishers, 1996), p. 19.

Christians stand at a juncture, and it is inextricable to this juncture that derivative bioethical stances are prescribed, assumed, and brought to bear with confident expectation into society for they carry both the imprimatur of divine truth and the promise of future fulfillment.

But therein again is the realism.

The new age is not yet fully come. The church still awaits the consummation of its hope in the glorious return of its Lord. Even though the ends of the ages have overlapped, the power of the old age still persists.

The Cross of Christ

Hence, Christians are moved to the second action frame, the cross of Christ. "The sufferings of this present time" will inevitably include frustrated bioethical imperatives, as well as ungodly cultural contradictions to passionate hearts for Christ's glory. And yet, here is the tension again: the redemptive power of the cross of Christ is still operative and remains so, ever incapable of being ultimately overthrown. It is this perspective that infuses the church's bioethical challenges, failures, and successes with an undying certainty of hope which validates needful mutual encouragement. Such encouragement rises out of the Christian common commendable identification with the Lord and the suffering of his crucifixion. Christians suffer together. Christians suffer doing bioethics together with confident expectation of making a difference.

Those who trust in Christ have the Holy Spirit. He indwells the believer and the collectivity of the believers called the church. He himself is termed the *arrabon,* a kind of earnest money already paid up front that guarantees unequivocally the full payment yet to follow. Hence, the failures experienced through the mockery of decaying cultural voices neither annihilate nor debilitate the bioethical action frame of the cross for intrusive intentional prophetic cultural guidance.

Up to this point, then, how do these first two action frames work together? What takes place under the intentionality of this theologically defined ecclesiastical identity? First, from the action frame of new creation identity, Christians gain confident expectation of bioethical efficacy. Second, they are also given sound basis for authentic and confident encouragement as a guiding norm for their bioethical failures, as well as triumphs, through the correlative action frame of the cross of Christ. This cross motivates the church to push on through all her points of societal ostracization rising from the specious icons of narcissistic hedonism and autonomous individualism whose end is the self and whose perpetuity is personal peace and affluence.

229

The cross, in contradistinction to the self-fulfillment motif of culture, is the divine moment of stamping human bioethical behavior with the validation of the joyful foolishness of self-sacrifice and the biblically celebrated foolishness of loving obedience to God even to the point of death. This is the foolishness of the cross over against the wisdom of the world — even to the point of death. But not a death into an arched oblivion of some nihilistic void of meaninglessness. Rather a death of suffering that is redeemed and certified eternal by virtue of the resurrection of Christ, the first fruits, the elder brother, from the dead. If Jesus' death were merely accidental, some mishap of a divine nap, some cosmic "oops!", then nothing is modeled worth emulating.

The Encouragement of the Cross

But in fact, his is not a death of mistake. His death is not a death of a stampeding conquering injustice against some *Übermensch* who tried valiantly, desperately to go for all the gusto and somehow in the midst of his self-serving pleasure, people sneaked up on him and crucified him. No, his death is rather that of the divine-human life willingly, freely, intentionally laid down for the benefit of others.

Hence, even though as the God-Man, Christ's death is unrepeatable and *sui generis*, still, for the faithful disciple who adores his Lord, the way of his death becomes the norm of behavior in bioethical persistence of the church into society. At times, and in fact due to the prevailing cultural winds, more often than not, this naturally requires confident mutual encouragement for this attitude that was in Christ to also be in his church (Phil. 2:6-11).

Truly, encouragement needs to be at the heart of the ecclesiastical bioethical enterprise. For just as Christ humbled himself (Phil. 2:8) and took the form of a slave, so the Philippians should in humility (2:3) become servants of the interests of others in the context of an obedience to the norm of the cross for the glory of God. It is this that counteracts the infusion of narcissistic hedonism into the church, and makes a holy people persistent to keep pushing forward for holy bioethical norms even though rejected or ostracized by others.

Cultural eclectic tolerationism inevitably breeds moral mediocrity. But moral mediocrity is overcome in the church by an ethical excellence arising from bioethical absolutes spurred onward by confident encouragement derived from the action frame and realism of the acceptable way of the cross.

Often, admittedly, it is at this juncture of suffering to the point of the cross when the action frame of confident encouragement needs to link with confident endurance. Times can get tough. So now the third action frame, community, needs to come into focus.

The Redeemed Community

The third action frame of New Testament community confronts the church in the context of grace and truth with this fact: Expectation and anticipation of imminent consummation cannot lead to abandonment of social responsibility. The culture must be impacted by bioethical ecclesiastical salt and light that has a unified voice. The church understands that such efforts to persuade and dissuade may result in its experiencing both suffering and joy paradoxically present until Christ's return. In the unity of community, the church gains the New Testament validated strength both to withstand and aggress under this eternal perspective.

From the Pauline perspective, the interdependent nature of Christian with Christian as the dwelling or temple of the Holy Spirit provides the fodder for keeping on in the face of seemingly insurmountable obstacles (1 Cor. 6:19-20). Just so, the intentionality of this community identity must be existentially embraced under the aegis of the preciousness of the mutuality of edification. This is done, once again, upon the basis of biblical authority defining the Christian with both a balanced spirituality and an objective basis for moral absolutes in the context of cherishing community.

Do Christians, however, adequately cherish church community?

One telling indictment rises from the joke about the Christian who was the only survivor of a shipwreck. He was washed up onto an island never inhabited by anyone. He was the first and only person on the island. Ten years passed before he was rescued. When the captain of the vessel came onto the island, this Christian proudly said, "Before I go with you, let me show you what I've accomplished these past ten years. Over here is the home I've built for myself. And over there is my church that I've built." The captain was impressed, and pointed to a third building and said, "What, sir, is that building there?"

The Christian answered, "Oh, that's the church I used to go to."

American individualism inculcated into the American church should be so lampooned as to show its risible inappropriateness.

For the first point for the establishment of endurance through the community is the valuation of the Bible's supernatural identity of the community itself. Here the culture's reductive naturalism and autonomous individualism are dismissed with a mere cursory glance by virtue of Paul's audacious metaphor in 1 Corinthians 3:16. Not only is the church God's building (3:10), having thereby supernatural origin. But its upkeep is maintained by the church being God's supernatural dwelling: "Do you not know that you [plural] are God's temple and that God's Spirit dwells in you [plural]?" (3:16). Admittedly, at a later juncture, this first expressed plural is inclusive of the latter expressed singular in 1 Corinthians 6:19. But to read here in 3:16 the singular is to miss the impact of the bold metaphor. The apostolic founded community in the plurality of its persons takes the place of the Jewish temple as the locus where the glory of God dwells. Body-wise, in the collectivity of their gathered physical presence, Christians have replaced the Jewish temple.

Reason for Endurance

Where the glory of God dwells, there is reason for endurance in doing bioethics in the face of all odds. "If God is for us, who can be against us?" (Rom. 8:31). Where the dwelling of God is, is the place for the validation of the believers' humble but sure entitlement to have faith in the future grace of all that God promises to be for them in Christ Jesus as Christian bioethics impact cultural positions.

Hence, the gathered community builds itself up to endurance with such edifying truths. The noun, *oikodome* ("building up," "edification"), and the cognate verb, *oikodomein*, occur repeatedly in the twelfth chapter of 1 Corinthians. That is, Paul who was used by God to lay the supernatural foundation in Jesus Christ, now recognizes that building maintenance is transferred to the human Christian community itself.

Moreover, it is imperative that community-building be an egalitarian distributed task in the moments of worship: "When you come together, each one has a hymn, or a word of instruction, a revelation, a tongue or an interpretation. All of these must be done for the strengthening of the church" (14:26). Intelligent prophesying builds up the church (14:3), whereas tongues is valuable but does not edify the community. *Simply, edification to the point of endurance intentionally comes in the context of the participatory mutuality of spirituality.*

The circular movement could be cited and summed this way: From the presence of the Holy Spirit comes the community which is called to mutual edification which in turn produces the confidence of mutual endurance traceable back to the origin of the Spirit who has called the temple into existence in the first place.

One other reinforcing passage worthy of citation before summation is

Romans 12:1-2: "Therefore, I urge you, brothers, in view of God's mercy, to offer your bodies as living sacrifices, holy and pleasing to God — this is your spiritual act of worship. Do not conform any longer to the pattern of this world, but be transformed by the renewing of your mind" (NIV).

This tends to be a focused favorite in the Christian community, but once again, usually with individualistic application. And yet, this is plural terminology and emphasis. It is the community conjointly that is to offer itself or themselves up as a living sacrifice, not the great American individual.

And with regard to the quality of a confident endurance, Paul's thought moves in Romans 12:2 from the community's sacrificial self-surrender to the community's transformation.

In light of this passage, from where does the community's freedom from the persuasive cultural voice come? Having offered themselves to God, community members are to find themselves transformed, set free from the confining power of this age. Their mind ("your bodies" is, obviously, the plural, but "mind" is, interestingly, the singular) is to be made new by God so that they can rightly discern God's will over against the confusions of a culture's heyday of multiple bioethical inducements and bioethical siren voices deceptively carrying mod rot.

Interconnected Action Frames for Bioethics

In summary, then, this is full circle back around to the action frames of new creation and cross. For the meaning of this Romans 12 apostolic and inspired vision is substantially the same as the picture of the church in 2 Corinthians 5:14-21 (above), in which the church, as new creation in Christ, is said to become "the righteousness of God." The only difference is that in 2 Corinthians 5, the new creation is affirmed as explosively current though bounded by the juncture of the already and the not yet, whereas in Romans 12, the concept is the continual conjoint offering up of ourselves in order in the future to become transformed together.

But, here again is the juncture of the already and the not yet, the indicative with the imperative, the exhortation to be now in Christ what surely we shall become at his return. From this comes the substance of faithful endurance.

For the constant factor through both and more is that the apostle via divine inspiration sees God's salvific work in corporate terms. That is, God transforms a people, not atomized individuals, to be a people of mutual expectation, encouragement, and endurance in doing bioethics. Consequently, from this, the people of God have ethical impact from the self-conscious identity as making a bioethical difference through new creation in collision with the present age (the *kosmos*), and cross as a paradigm for encouraging action to the point of suffering sacrifice, with their concomitant inescapable manifestation in the world as the body of Christ, the community of God, keeping on, keeping on, thereby both impeding and altering the progress of mod rot by the Christian presentation and infusion of a biblical bioethical freshness into the cultural scene.

Christian Teaching and the Church's Authority

Marsha D. Fowler, Ph.D.

Social Ethics and Faith Communities

Spiritual longings, not unlike biological urges and emotional needs, indicate to us an aspect of our essential created nature — that we were created to live in relationship. "I" becomes "we" in couples, families, and communities. Who "we" are, then, becomes an aspect of our shared history and experiences, our traditions, our story or narrative, our identity. Within our Christian communities, "we" hear God speak to Moses, saying to us as well:

> Go and assemble the elders of Israel, and say to them, "The Lord, the God of your ancestors, the God of Abraham, of Isaac, and of Jacob, has appeared to me, saying: 'I have given heed to you and to what has been done to you in Egypt. I declare that I will bring you up out of the misery of Egypt, to the land of the Canaanites, the Hittites, the Amorites, the Perizzites, the Hivites, and the Jebusites, a land flowing with milk and honey.'" They will listen to your voice; and you and the elders of Israel shall go to the king of Egypt and say to him, "The Lord, the God of the Hebrews, has met with us; let us now go a three days' journey into the wilderness, so that we may sacrifice to the Lord our God." I know, however, that the king of Egypt will not let you go unless compelled by a mighty hand. So I will stretch out my hand and strike Egypt with all my wonders that I will perform in it; after that he will let you go. (Exod. 3:16-20)

In the book of the Acts of the Apostles, the Gentile Luke says that "the God of Abraham, the God of Isaac, and the God of Jacob, the God of our ancestors has glorified his servant Jesus . . ." (Acts 3:13) so our shared story, as Christians, stretches back into the land of Ur of the Chaldees.

And yet, as Christians we nonetheless have diverse stories, stories that arise from historical contexts of great moment, such as the Protestant Reformation or, as in my own story, from a man named Calvin in the theocracy of Geneva and from John Knox the firebrand who blew "The First Blast of the Trumpet against the Monstrous Regiment of Women."

John Calvin, the brilliant systematizer; John Knox, both hagiographized and vilified; Scots grey; cold and damp Edinburgh; black wool preaching robes; Genevan Psalter; Heidelberg and Westminster catechisms; Scots' Confession; clans and kilts and haggis; St. Giles, High Kirk of Scotland; John Knox buried under parking space 44; all the way to America, and more particularly to California: my own tradition. Yet a tradition is more than specific and right beliefs and historical events. It is a mindset, a worldview, an interpretive lens, a culture. My understanding, then, of my responsibilities toward God, myself, and neighbor, will be shaped, informed, and colored by this faith culture. Stanley Hauerwas has written that "the form and substance of a community is narrative dependent and therefore what counts as 'social ethics' is a correlative of that narrative."[1] The form and substance of my community, of your community, cannot be separated from the narrative of that community.

Hauerwas also writes that "every social ethics involves a narrative, whether it is concerned with the formulation of basic principles of social organization or concrete policy alternatives."[2] If a church, in the broader denominational sense, is going to "create" a social ethics, its members must know their shared narrative that gives structure, coherence, and boundaries to that social ethics. Without this, a social ethics becomes as those who shoot wildly, frantically, aimlessly into the darkness and are as likely to shoot themselves as anything else. And so, the aberrations, idiosyncrasies, distinctives, and character of a tradition become both intrinsic and essential to the formulation of a social ethics. In this conceptualization, a social ethics is not created as such, but it emerges from the tradition to be renewed to fit the exigencies of the day.

Perhaps a more specific example might be useful from the tradition that has shaped my own perspectives. If one is to look at the formulation of a

---

1. Stanley Hauerwas, *A Community of Character: Toward a Constructive Christian Social Ethic* (Notre Dame: Notre Dame University Press, 1981), p. 9.
2. Hauerwas, *Community of Character*, p. 10.

Christian social ethics the question that arises immediately is: What is the relationship of spiritual concerns to temporal concerns? This is, of course, a question that must be asked about one's own particular tradition, and the answer will vary from one tradition to another. In my own Reformed/Presbyterian understanding, our *Book of Order* (Constitution, Part II Presbyterian Church [USA]) identifies the "Great Ends of the Church" as

- the proclamation of the gospel for the salvation of humankind
- the shelter, nurture, and spiritual fellowship of the children of God
- the maintenance of divine worship
- the preservation of the truth
- the promotion of social righteousness
- and the exhibition of the Kingdom of Heaven to the world[3]

Thus, a responsibility and mandate for social transformation and work toward social justice is intrinsic to a Presbyterian understanding of the role of the church. Such a mandate arises, not from the *Book of Order* itself, but from the theology of the Reformed tradition from the 1500s to the present. Contemporary statements, such as the *Confession of 1967*, renew this charge:

> In each time and place there are particular problems and crises through which God calls the church to act. The church, guided by the Spirit, humbled by its own complicity and instructed by all attainable knowledge, seeks to discern the will of God and learn how to obey in these concrete situations.[4]

The church, then, must act, not by its own desires or design, not blindly or capriciously, not from ignorance or untutored understanding, but in discernment and obedience to the Word of God.

A rather more direct statement can be found in the recent Brief Statement of Faith (written to celebrate the 1983 reunion of the United Presbyterian Church in the USA and the Presbyterian Church in the US), which expresses the major themes of the Reformed faith.

> In a broken and fearful world
> the Spirit gives us courage

---

3. Presbyterian Church (USA), *The Book of Order 1999-2000*, Constitution, part II (Louisville, Ky.: Presbyterian Church [USA]), §G-1.0200.
4. PC(USA), *The Book of Confessions*, Constitution, part I (Louisville, Ky.: Presbyterian Church [USA]), §9.43.

to pray without ceasing,
to witness among all peoples to Christ as Lord and Savior,
to unmask idolatries in Church and culture,
to hear the voices of peoples long silenced,
and to work with others for justice, freedom, and peace.[5]

The theology of this tradition maintains that there is a "human tendency toward tyranny and idolatry"[6] that manifests itself both within and outside the church. Thus, transformation is not simply "social" but always, at one and the same time, ecclesiastical. The watchword of the Reformed tradition that asserts this is *ecclesia reformata, semper reformanda,* that is, "the church reformed, always being reformed according to the Word of God and the call of the Spirit."[7] In this there is, as an inescapable part of Reformed theology, a demand for "reform."

What Is Social Ethics?

Perhaps, however, a discussion of social ethics as social transformation or reformation through the work of the church is premature until the question of "what is social ethics?" has been addressed. Gibson Winter defines social ethics as "issues of social order — the good, right, and ought in the organization of human communities and the shaping of social policies. Hence the subject matter of social ethics is moral rightness in the shaping of human society."[8] For Winter,

> Ethical analysis takes place in order to approve and strengthen those institutions or aspects of a sector of the social system that sustain moral community, and in order to criticize, transform, or undermine those institutions or aspects of the social system that destroy such possibilities.[9]

The church is not exempt, of course, from ethical analysis. In fact, that is the starting point of Christian social ethics.

---

5. PC(USA), *Book of Confessions* §10.4, lines 65-71.
6. PC(USA), *Book of Order,* §G-2.0500.
7. PC(USA), *Book of Order,* §G-2.0200.
8. Gibson Winter, *Elements for a Social Ethics* (New York: Macmillan, 1966), p. 215.
9. Winter, *Social Ethics,* p. 215.

The Functions of Social Ethics

Social ethics has three essential moral functions: (1) reform within, (2) epidictic discourse, and (3) the reform of society. Social ethics has an intrinsic reformist bias that contends for change within a given community, seeking to bring the *is* into conformity with the *ought*. It actively and participatorily embraces the notion "thy kingdom come, thy will be done, on earth as it is in heaven," both within the *ecclesia* and outside it. Within the church, reform requires critical self-reflection and evaluation and a commitment to obedient follow-through. Both responsiveness to the promptings of the Holy Spirit and "ears to hear" are necessary to accomplish this.

The ears that hear are attuned to God's voice as heard in Scripture read and proclaimed, as heard in the fellowship of the community, as heard — and tasted — in the sacrament of the Lord's Supper, as heard in the sound like the sudden rush of a violent wind from heaven (Acts 2:2). The language we speak and hear by which we may be led to action is of a particular sort: it is *epidictic discourse*. Epidictic (meaning "to show") discourse

> sets out to increase the intensity of adherence to certain values, which might not be contested when considered on their own, but may nevertheless not prevail against other values that might come into conflict with them.[10]

The function of epidictic discourse is to remind the hearers of their shared values and value structure in order to "increase the intensity of adherence to values held in common by the audience and the speaker . . . making use of dispositions already present in the audience" in order to foster action upon those values.[11] Epidictic discourse reminds the group of the *ought* in contrast to the *is* in its own communal life, as well as in the society that it seeks to influence. Such language is often heard in relation to support of mission endeavors, or stewardship drives, or in arguments over ministry *versus* business values in the operations of the church. It is common in Scripture and in preaching, often having a hortatory or a paranetic impetus. Epidictic discourse, then, brings together the need and movement toward reform within the group with the evocation of the group's values to overcome inertia where it exists and to galvanize to action.

The third function of social ethics is to represent the perspectives of the

10. C. Perlman and L. Olbrechts-Tyteca, *The New Rhetoric: A Treatise on Argumentation* (Notre Dame: Notre Dame University Press, 1969), p. 51.

11. Perlman and Olbrechts-Tyteca, *New Rhetoric*, pp. 52-53.

community to the larger society.[12] This function, still using epidictic discourse, but this time upon society itself, argues for change in society in accord with the moral norms of the community. Here, social ethics becomes an intrinsically political act.

To engage in social ethics is not without danger:

> As he [Jesus] came near and saw the city, he wept over it. . . . Then he entered the temple and began to drive out those who were selling things there; and he said, "It is written, 'My house shall be a house of prayer'; but you have made it a den of robbers." Every day he was teaching in the temple. The chief priests, the scribes, and the leaders of the people kept looking for a way to kill him; but they did not find anything they could do, for all the people were spellbound by what they heard.[13]

Jesus himself, and more than a few saints over the centuries, have been martyred for speaking to society in ways that expose and condemn injustices and inhumanities, or in today's lexicon, for "political incorrectness." It is dangerous to challenge in any arena, even within the church. The church itself has martyred its own who spoke out of season. 'Tis a perilous thing "to challenge the social and political idols of men and women — more dangerous than to challenge individual morality."[14] Idols such as prestige, power, and money fight back.

Moral Suasion

Moral and religious arguments are not always persuasive in society. In earlier times, when religion and morality were more closely aligned, the coercive force of *moral suasion* was stronger. In days before the printing press, when books were hand-copied, the scribes placed a curse or a blessing in the front of the book, a blessing that the reader might profit or a curse that the book

---

12. Perlman and Olbrechts-Tyteca, *New Rhetoric;* Marsha Fowler, "Social Ethics and Nursing," in N. L. Chaska, ed., *The Nursing Profession: The Turning Points* (St. Louis: Mosby, 1989), pp. 24-30.

13. B. Metzger and R. Murphy, eds., *The New Oxford Annotated Bible; the New Revised Standard Version with Apocryphal/Deuterocanonical Books* (New York: Oxford University Press, 1991). (All quotations from Scripture in this essay are taken from this version.)

14. Task Force on Why and How the Church Makes a Social Policy Witness, *Why and How the Church Makes a Social Policy Witness: A Background Paper for Churchwide Study and Discussion* (Louisville, Ky.: Presbyterian Church [USA], September 1989), p. 3.

thief might perish. Witness the following inscription placed, by the copyist, in an ancient book:

> For him that stealeth, or borroweth and returneth not, this book from its owner, let it change into a serpent in his hand and rend him. Let him be struck with palsy, and all his members blasted. Let him languish in pain crying aloud for mercy, and let there be no surcease to his agony till he sing in dissolution. Let bookworms gnaw his entrails in token of the Worm that dieth not and when at last he doth go to his final punishment, let the flames of Hell consume him forever.[15]

When curses were believed to be a performative utterance (that is, that it would surely come to pass), and when moral infractions were dark sins, such a curse would likely dissuade those who were tempted. Not today.

A more communal example of moral action that encompasses all three functions of social ethics is found in the example of the village of Eyam, England, in the 1660s when the Great Plague raged through Europe. In September 1665 a tailor received a bolt of cloth that was infested with the fleas that carried the plague. When the pestilence remitted months later, seventy-seven were dead. Then, in the late spring of 1666 the plague broke out again in the tiny village. The rich had already left, and now the commonfolk, although with nowhere to go, also decided to flee the village. Their village rector, twenty-eight-year-old William Mompesson, exhorted the villagers to quarantine themselves to protect the people of surrounding Derbyshire from the spread of the plague. His words and position were persuasive and the villagers agreed. The town was marked out by a circle of white-painted stones in a half-mile radius as a warning to keep away. Provisions and goods that the village needed were left outside the perimeter of the stones. When the plague finally remitted, 259 of the 350 villagers were dead. This community united and determined to risk their own lives for the sake of others. This heroic act is celebrated each year in the English Midlands in the same field in which young Rector Mompesson preached.

Against Quietism

Christians are called to be the salt of the earth and the light of the world (Matt. 5:13-14). Characteristically this requires action and rejects quietism.

---

15. Marc Drogin, *Anathema! Medieval Scribes and the History of Book Curses* (Totowa, N.J.: Allanheld, Osmun, & Co. Publishers, 1983), p. 88.

Quietism, the removal from the world and worldly concerns to become immersed in God, free of the world or any of its claims or needs, is tantamount to the desalinization of the world and is morally and theologically unacceptable. Congregations that are solely inward looking, without reaching outward, are living in a way that is inconsistent with the gospel.

> God calls the church to be distinct from the structures that enslave people (although the church can become such a structure itself) and as a body with a voice to confront structures on behalf of people who are being harmed by existing social policies. . . .[16]

The church is a *body* — that *acts* — with *voice*. It *confronts* — on *behalf* of those being harmed by existing policies. Each of these key terms is important. The church is a *body*, being united, working together, not alone. It exercises social *voice*, speaks out prophetically, does not let pass without notice that which is harmful or unjust. It is a voice that attempts to speak God's words. The church *confronts*, that is, exercises voice with action. It does so on *behalf of* persons who have no voice.

Faith and life, then, whether individually or collectively, may not be separated. Faith critiques life personally, in community, or in the *polis*. Arthur Simon writes,

> The separation of religion from life contradicts the Biblical witness and therefore the Christian understanding of faith. To take major areas of life, those having to do with social and economic decisions that vitally affect all of us, and put them into a compartment carefully separated from faith is to turn much of life over to the devil.[17]

Metaphorically, quietism causes the desalinization of the world, as we said, giving much of life over to the prince of the low salt world, the ruler of the no salt kingdom.

So far, the role of tradition in social ethics, the nature and functions of social ethics, and the quietistic rejection of social ethics have been discussed in brief, all of which concludes that the church has a gospel obligation to work in the world to transform it. Yet, the questions of *how to do so* and *what difference* the church ought to make have not been addressed. How is it that the church engages in salt-loading and light therapy?

---

16. PC(USA) Task Force, *Social Policy Witness.*
17. Arthur Simon, *Christian Faith and Public Policy: No Grounds for Divorce* (Grand Rapids: Eerdmans, 1988), p. 12.

This has not been easy in recent years. The religious voice has been silenced in the public arena, more specifically the Christian voice has been muted in public life, sometimes by nuances of the law, sometimes by political correctness, sometimes by pluralistic concern, often by trivialization and other reasons.[18] One of those other reasons is "risk." 'Tis a fearful thing to fall into the hands of the living God — for God may call us to take the risk of speaking. But even more, 'tis a dangerous thing to place our lives in the hands of our legislators without participation in the political process. Yet, we have much to learn from legislators.

Social Compromise

Legislation, by its very nature, involves compromise. Indeed, legislators are about making compromises to the end that good legislation is produced. Not all compromise is good, of course. Compromise that violates one's integrity or faith is not a good compromise. But those compromises that do in fact maintain one's faith and integrity can be good compromises, amortizing particular interests and serving the common good. The rub is that many Christians view any compromise at all as intrinsically, by nature, by definition, in essence — wrong. Yet, social ethics requires social action, and social action requires political action, and political action requires negotiation, and negotiation requires compromise. How then, in seeking to transform society, can the church effect social change without compromising the values of the faith tradition?

Social Power Structures, and Social Meaning and Value Structures

Social institutions, including society as a whole, are comprised of structures that preserve and rectify (or destroy) the moral ethos of society. These include structures of social power, and structures of meaning and value.[19] Structures of social power include all the various forms of power that one sees in society: legal authority, position, coercive force, money, prestige, and

18. Stephen Carter, *The Culture of Disbelief: How American Law and Politics Trivialize Religious Belief* (New York: Harper Collins, 1993).
19. Max Stackhouse, "Ethics: Social and Christian," *Andover Newton Quarterly* 13 (1973): 173-91.

so on. Power structures have the capacity to "implement," that is, the power to act toward the realization of the community's values, meaning, and goals. Meaning and value structures, sometimes capsulized as "ethics," set boundaries, such as what constitutes legitimate means or ends, inform and critique power structures, and reshape power structures in accord with the community's values and meaning.

It is possible for power structures to overwhelm meaning and values structures and to engage in run-away self-interest. It is also possible, though less often the case, that meaning and value structures can immobilize power structures. The implications of the relationship between power structures and meaning and value structures for the socially transforming church is that what must be sought is a balance in which power structures inform meaning and value structures and live out those values in the real world; and meaning and value structures that critique power structures and reshape them in accord with the value of the community. While it is rarely the case that meaning and value structures render power structures impotent, it is the case that power structures can and do leave the meaning and value structures behind in the dust of demise. In the view set forth here, power structures and meaning and value structures (or ethics) must be maintained in dynamic, social equilibrium with one another. To realize this tension, the church both acts within and outside the power structures to transform them, but does so by embracing, implementing, and proclaiming its meaning and central values, recognizing the plurality of values socially held.

Asserting Meaning and Value Structures

Wisdom and discernment are a part of this task. We must recognize that false gods or idols have a seductive power that moves toward their adoption in the arena of political negotiation (that human tendency toward tyranny and idolatry), rather than toward the affirmation or reaffirmation of the meaning and value structures that are life-giving for all. But, what might be one such value that the church would seek to affirm?

The ancient concept of *shalom* would serve as a good example here. *Shalom* is usually, rather inadequately, translated into English as "peace." However, *shalom* has a

> . . . wide semantic range stressing various meanings of its basic meaning: totality or completeness. These meanings include fulfillment, completion, maturity, soundness, wholeness (both individual and communal), commu-

nity, harmony, tranquility, security, well-being, welfare, friendship, agreement, success, prosperity.[20]

Shalom seeks the good of the individual as well as the community; and seeks the good of the community as well as the individual. They are inseparable. What might a ministry and mission that seeks shalom look like? It would be a ministry (to those within the church) and a mission (to those outside the church) that is incarnational, transfigurative, transformative, prophetic.[21]

Seeking Shalom in Ministry and Mission

A ministry and mission that is incarnational embraces the whole of life, on good days or evil days, in health or in brokenness, and reclaims the belief that life will inevitably entail some degree of suffering — and that we are called to mitigate one another's suffering through personal caring, by the individual or the community for another or others, and through the social changes that may be needed. We are to bring our selves and God into the presence of those who suffer. An incarnational ministry and mission, for example, seeks to comfort and provide for those who have suffered from natural disaster, or works to make the environment accessible to those who are energy or mobility limited, or seeks to prevent the suffering that drunk driving causes. Personal caring and social transformation.

A transformative ministry and mission changes us from what we were to what we ought to be. It looks inside the walls of the church and demands that its own unfairnesses or injustices or neglectful behavior be changed. It also looks outward, toward the community and demands those same changes. It always picks up the man beaten by thieves on the road to Jericho, binds up his wounds and cares for him. That is, it does the unexpected, the unrequired, and sets a new definition of who is our neighbor. Personal change and social witness.

Transfiguration is the illumination of our lives that occurs in the encounter with the living God. In that encounter we find that our lives are fragmented, our priorities are deranged, and that our souls are dry. In transfiguration we dip into the living water of the well of God, seeking to restore and

20. R. F. Youngblood, "Peace," in *The International Standard Bible Encyclopedia*, ed. G. Bromily, rev. ed., vol. 3 (Grand Rapids: Eerdmans, 1986), p. 732.

21. Fowler, "The Church as a Welcoming Community," in *Genetic Ethics: Do the Ends Justify the Genes?* ed. J. Kilner, R. Pentz, and F. Young (Grand Rapids: Eerdmans, 1997), pp. 246-55.

renew our lives in accord with the will of God; therein lies the abundant life that has been promised us. A ministry and mission that is transfigurative is in communion with God to the end of the reprioritization and renewal of values, personal, communal, and social. Personal obedience and social renewal.

A ministry and mission that is prophetic speaks or proclaims in the name of God. It proclaims that God seeks for us to be healed, to be whole, both as individuals, as congregations, as a society. Thus the prophetic voice calls for repentance and change, pronounces a warning, and denounces that which is destructive of human health or dignity and proclaims that which affirms the *imago dei* and human community; personal repentance and social healing.

In these attributes of a ministry and mission of shalom, the church seeks, within itself and for society, a *telos* of shalom — totality or completeness — over against *teloi* that deprive, enslave, or perpetrate and perpetuate injustice and privilege. It does so through social witness and social witness policies.

Social Witness and Social Witness Policies

Social witness and social witness policies are a part of the "how" of the transformation of society by the church. Social witness is the witness of the church to society — local, state, national, and international. Social witness policies are policies that, in their formulation, proclaim the gospel as understood by the particular tradition, and as it impinges upon society, asserting gospel values in relation to specific issues. Social witness and social witness policies can arise from local congregations, regional judicatories, or national denominations. Examples of faith- and church-related local social witness, cases that have had a profound impact upon the Los Angeles metropolitan area, include:

- Project Angel: a project that provides layettes for newborn babies whose families cannot afford the necessities for infant care
- Union Station: a project that centralizes resources to assist homeless persons and families by providing shelter, food, and counseling
- The Mary Magdalene Project: a residential and counseling project that takes in women who are working as prostitutes who wish to leave that lifestyle, helping them to transition into a new life
- Door of Hope: a residential project that assists nuclear families who have suffered a reversal of circumstances to transition into a new life

In each of these endeavors a specific social need or social ill was "targeted for extinction" and local action was taken to realize that goal. While these projects are rather "large," the premise in social witness is that any church, however large or small, however wealthy or poor, has the capacity to reach out to the community that surrounds it to seek its *shalom*. The health ministry within my own small church offers aerobics classes, walking groups, and free blood pressure screening to its members as well as to community residents. Social witness, then, models the values of the faith including values of justice and health.

Social witness policy functions at a different level. In social witness policy the church (whether a denomination, or a local or regional ecumenical council) formulates a statement that critiques an aspect of society and calls for change arguing on the basis of meaning and value structures. The process of formulating a social witness policy includes:

- Examining Scripture, creeds and confessions, and theological works for greater Christian understanding and guidance
- Soliciting special insights from those persons who are affected by the problem or issue; hearing their stories; discovering what *is*
- Soliciting the special insights from experts who have studied the issue and have worked in the field
- Seeking the wisdom of ecumenical dialogue and modeling Christian collaboration in a way that combines the resources of "time, talent, and treasure"
- Looking at the horizon to see the broader social context of the issue, related concerns, possibilities of amelioration or prevention, envisioning a desired future
- Pray, pray, pray
- Proclaiming what *ought* to be and urging its realization

Any issue or problem that potentially damages or undermines shalom is a fitting subject for a social witness policy. Whether the issue is the sale of tobacco near high or grade schools; illiteracy; domestic abuse; access to health care; elder neglect; drunk driving; animal mistreatment; ethnic discord; prostitution; substance abuse; hunger; poverty; or any number of social problems, all are likely to benefit from the collective voice of the church speaking out against the problem and seeking to resolve it through tangible action.

How Then Shall We Live?

How then shall we live as Christians concerned to transform society that "thy kingdom come, thy will be done on earth as it is in heaven"? In order to create a relevant social ethics that will seek the transformation of society in regard to particular issues specific steps are required. Each church or congregation must:

- Know your own particular faith tradition, its formative narrative, and the elements of its social ethics
- Engage in critical self-reflection and evaluation of the church and seek to "unmask the idolatries of the church" as you discern them
- Teach and preach patterns of meaning and value (moral and spiritual formation) for young and old
- Call the people, call each other, to embrace the values of the Christian tradition as it is particularly understood
- Assert and advance meaning and value structures; critique the status quo
- Reach out into society to "unmask idolatries of culture": speak prophetically, act decisively as the Spirit leads, seek God's shalom for all
- Shape and transform power structures from within and without; engage in the political process
- As a church, engage in social witness and formulate and adopt social witness policies

And yet, with all this, one thing remains: Pray for the *polis*, the city. As the prophet Jeremiah spoke, ". . . seek the welfare of the city where I [the LORD] have sent you into exile, and pray to the LORD on its behalf, for in its welfare you will find your welfare" (Jer. 29:7).

Pastoral Care in the Abortion Society

Terry A. Schlossberg, M.A.

The Christian church in America has been slow to respond to the moral and pastoral challenges of abortion. To a large extent, it was Catholic parishioners in community-based right-to-life organizations who formed the first formidable front of opposition to the legislative changes thrust upon the society following *Roe v. Wade* (1973). Catholic social services were the first form of ministry intervention for women who otherwise considered abortion their only option in a problem pregnancy. Protestant believers gradually joined in resisting the effects of the *Roe v. Wade* decision until they have become a force in their own right. But the institutional churches largely withheld moral comment until Pope John Paul II's *Evangelium Vitae (The Gospel of Life)*[1] in 1995. There are small evidences of churches seeking to give witness and to provide pastoral care in response to abortion. This organized activity remains a weak ministry, characterized by a perception of division and by pastors' avoidance of the subject. Consequently, the Christian response to abortion continues to take the form of individuals and groups of Christians who work in community-based and para-church organizations, with little teaching and leadership from churches.

After nullifying state laws restricting abortion not quite three decades ago, the United States has recorded more than 35 million abortions. More than one in four pregnancies ends in abortion, and women under the age of twenty-five are the most affected group.[2] Women who had abortions in the

1. Pope John Paul II, *Evangelium Vitae* (Boston: Pauline Books & Media, 1995).
2. "Facts in Brief" (New York and Washington: The Alan Guttmacher Institute, Jan. 1997).

1970s and 1980s are no longer young singles, but abortion remains a part of their personal histories. Though church membership has a deterring effect on abortion, nearly 20 percent of the women having abortions describe themselves as committed believers.[3] It is doubtful that there is a single established church in which abortion has not touched members' lives or been a factor in the youth group dynamic.

The Christian news magazine *World* summarized the findings of its own survey of the church's pastoral ministry on abortion in the title of a 1995 article: "Silence of the Shepherds."[4] The summary includes a statement by Billy Graham, whom the magazine describes as arguably the leader of American evangelicalism. On a late-night television show, host Larry King asked why Graham had not spoken to President Clinton regarding the President's views on abortion. Graham answered:

> Because my message is the gospel of Christ, which I think is the good news that God loves us, that Christ died on the cross for us, that he rose again and he's coming back again. And I don't get into these things like abortion and some of these other issues that people are involved in today. I feel like that's not my main message.

Then *World* puts this question to its readers: "Abortion and the gospel: unrelated matters?"

World did not single out Billy Graham to criticize him. His statement expresses publicly what the magazine surmises may be in the minds of thousands of American pastors, and what may explain the "silence" of the "shepherds." Abortion is often regarded as a diversion from the real mission of the church because it is thought to be more a controversial, social, and political issue than a matter of morality. Society, including pastors, moreover, tend to perceive moral issues as murky and confusing.

A statement by the Presbyterian Church in 1869, however, shows that the church was able, in its fairly recent history, to understand and express a relationship between the gospel and abortion:

> This Assembly regards the destruction by parents of their own offspring, before birth, with abhorrence, as a crime against God and against nature; and as the frequency of such murders can no longer be concealed, we

---

3. Reported by Frederica Matthews-Green in *Christianity Today*, April 7, 1997, p. 28. The statement is based on a 1996 survey by the Alan Guttmacher Institute in which 18 percent of women at abortion clinics responded with "yes" to the question, "Do you consider yourself a born-again Christian or Evangelical Christian?"

4. Joe Maxwell, "Silence of the Shepherds," *World*, January 21, 1995, pp. 12-17.

hereby warn those that are guilty of this crime that, except they repent, they cannot inherit eternal life. . . .[5]

The church modeled a pastoral warning, connecting abortion with sin and calling the guilty to repentance and salvation. It is not a statement of public policy. The church made what is always the church's strongest appeal: her calling to bring the word of redemption to the culture.

God calls pastors in our age into a situation of great moral evil, where sin is not only practiced quietly and shamefully, but also trumpeted as a good. Churches need not enter the debate over what the law should be to fulfill their calling. But Christian churches cannot fully live out their calling in our time without speaking and ministering in response to the greatest moral problem of our time: legally sanctioned killing of the innocent.

The church is the institution called by God to speak the word of God into the surrounding culture, and to minister his provision to those in need and his grace to those who have fallen. In a country where there have been well over one million induced abortions every year for nearly three decades, each one a decision of choice, the need for the ministry of the Christian church ought to be obvious. If the church is to make a difference in both the numbers and effects of abortion on our society, we in our congregations shall have to develop strategies for a far more effectual ministry than currently exists.

Strategies for the Ministry of Preaching and Teaching

A first strategy for ending the church's silence on abortion is to help pastors rediscover the relationship between abortion and the teaching office to which they are called, and to recognize that the teaching office requires of pastors that they confront error and sin.

Gilbert Meilaender, a Lutheran professor of ethics, distinguishes between the church's role in teaching the biblical ethic and its role in the pastoral care of souls.[6] In stating the biblical ethic, he says, we are saying what the church's public teaching ought to be if it wishes to be faithful to Scripture. In pastoral care, we are asking what is the faithful practical application of the biblical ethic to members of the flock of God as each situation arises. The lat-

---

5. The Bills and Overtures Committee of the General Assembly of the Presbyterian Church in the United States, meeting in 1869.

6. Gilbert Meilaender, "The First of Institutions," *Pro Ecclesia* 6, no. 4 (Fall 1997): 444-56.

ter is the more difficult, says Meilaender, but is rendered impossible without clarity about the former.

> To articulate the Christian norm for life is not the church's only task, but it is a necessary task. If we fail here, affirmation of and compassion for those who fall short mean little. Indeed, once we can no longer say what it means to "fall short," we have little need for compassion and few problems for pastoral practice.[7]

Several years ago, I received a handwritten letter from a young woman that illustrates Meilaender's point. She said she finally understood why no one in the church had ever warned her away from abortion. It is because they do not really believe it is wrong, she said. She explained that she grew up in a church with no moral teaching. She wandered away as a teenager. She got pregnant and had an abortion. Only after her fourth abortion did she hit bottom and begin looking for help. Finally, after many years of living with her feelings of guilt and seeing multiple counselors who were not able to help her, someone led her to faith in Jesus Christ. She finally found forgiveness, restoration from her abortions and her sexual sin, and a process of healing, which she was in when she wrote the letter. She was filled with the regret of wishing someone in the church had steered her away from all that trouble in the first place.

The gospel is not for good people; Jesus said it was not to the righteous, but to sinners that he came (Luke 5:32). Implicit in the pastoral calling is resistance to the culture's attempt to reconstruct or redefine sin so that people become good by definition. The pastoral calling is rather to speak the truth into the culture's denial. It is to bring that great stumbling block that Jesus is to confront those ideologies that take people captive, that dress the wound of God's people as if the sins do not matter (Jer. 8:11). It is to confront that which calls evil good, and good evil (Isa. 5:20). There is no more important example of the need to counter the prevailing cultural norms today than this area of abortion. If the confrontation of truth against falsehood does not come from the pastoral office of the church, we cannot expect to see it come from anywhere else. This necessary aspect of the teaching role of the pastor was modeled by the Presbyterian Church in 1869 when it spoke a clear biblical ethic into the culture on the subject of abortion: an unequivocal "Thou shalt not. . . ."

There is no getting around it. Telling the truth about abortion sooner or later requires the negative message that the modern church is so reluctant to proclaim. It is necessary in helping people recognize error when they meet it. Jesus himself showed the power of the negative in his denunciations of evil. It

---

7. Meilaender, "The First of Institutions," p. 455.

was he who accused false teachers of being "ravening wolves" and "blind guides," terms that offend our sensitivities today. This avoidance of the negative and insistence on the positive is at the heart of what Dietrich Bonhoeffer calls "cheap grace." Pastors will need to find the courage to overcome their reticence, and to call abortion a sin.

Historical Teachings of the Church as a Strategy

The message is much more than the negative, however. There is a wealth of positive biblical teaching that lays the groundwork for the "Thou shalt not" of abortion. Teaching about the unborn and about God's value for us before we were born is itself seldom expressed in the church today. Restoring that teaching is valuable in itself, and makes opposition to abortion a logical conclusion even when the negative is left unspoken.

Seminaries do not provide training in preaching and teaching on abortion in a biblical and pastoral framework. That means that in order for this strategy of giving good, effective public moral witness to work, pastors will need to have opportunities to learn how to proclaim the message about abortion in the context of the Christian gospel. Good model sermons are an effective help. In an effort to demonstrate good preaching within a Christian spiritual and theological framework, our organization published in 1995 a collection of ten sermons preached by mainline Presbyterians on abortion.[8]

Drawing on the breadth of doctrines of the Christian church to show how life-affirming they are is a strategy for developing and teaching the biblical ethic on life.[9] The obvious place to begin is where the Bible itself begins: with the doctrine of creation and God's forming of human beings in his own image (Gen. 1:27). God is the one who forms us (Ps. 139:13-16), and the one who gives meaning to our lives (Jer. 1:5; Gal. 1:15). This teaching is rejected by modern ideologies that assert there is nothing distinctive about being human. Peter Singer, for example, repudiates the Judeo-Christian ethic

---

8. *Fearfully and Wonderfully Made: A Collection of Sermons on Life by Presbyterians* (Burke, Va.: Presbyterians Pro-Life, Research, Education, and Care, Inc., 1995). For an ecumenical collection, see Paul T. Stallsworth, ed., *The Right Choice* (Nashville: Abingdon Press, 1997).

9. In 1996 our organization published an apologetic for our position on abortion called "A Firm Foundation: Christian Theology and Abortion" (Burke, Va.: Presbyterians Pro-Life, Research, Education, and Care, Inc., 1996). The booklet lays out the rationale for what the church has always believed and taught about abortion life from Scripture, using the historic doctrines of Christian faith.

as the primary hindrance to acceptance of a more up-to-date ethic for making life and death decisions.[10] Singer's appointment as ethics professor at Princeton University shows that rejection of the Christian teaching on the distinctives of humanness and the implications of such teaching are no longer simply expressions of an extremist fringe element in the society. The church needs to respond out of its own doctrines to this rejection of the biblical worldview.

God's sovereignty — his ownership of the world — is a teaching in conflict with the assertion of the complete autonomy of women to make their own decisions about their own bodies. Our belonging to God means that we are not our own, but rather were bought with a price (1 Cor. 6:19, 20). A Catholic organization called Priests for Life has a pamphlet that draws a vivid visual contrast between worldviews with two pictures. The first is of women marching with placards that read, "It's my body!," the classic expression of radical feminist autonomy. The second picture on the pamphlet is of the crucified Christ saying, "This is my body, given for you . . . ," the ultimate expression of love. We belong to God, and that belonging has implications for how we live. One of the Christian church's most familiar professions of faith comes from the opening to the sixteenth-century Heidelberg Catechism, which asks, "What is your only comfort in life and in death?" and answers:

> My only comfort in life and in death is that I belong — body and soul — not to myself but to my faithful Savior, Jesus Christ, who at the cost of his own blood has fully paid for all my sins and has completely freed me from the dominion of the devil; that he protects me so well that without the will of my Father in heaven not a hair can fall from my head; indeed, that everything must fit his purpose for my salvation. Therefore, by his Holy Spirit, he also assures me of eternal life, and makes me wholeheartedly willing and ready from now on to live for him.[11]

In this affirmation of the church's teaching we see the whole of the Christian life integrated into the belonging to God, which is the antithesis of abortion doctrine. In every doctrine of the Christian church pastors can find a message regarding the preservation and nurture of human life that can be positively and effectively applied to build a pro-life consensus in the church.

---

10. Peter Singer's explicit rejection of the Judeo-Christian ethic is found in an editorial in *The Journal of Pediatrics* (July 1983), but see also his book *Practical Ethics*, 2nd ed. (Cambridge: Cambridge University Press, 1993).

11. *The Heidelberg Catechism, 1563* (Grand Rapids: CRC Publications, 1988), p. 9.

Strategies for Pastoral Care: The Body's Commitment to Children and to Its Corporate Unity as a Forgiven People

Areas related to the church's sacramental life bring us across the threshold from preaching and teaching into pastoral care ministry. But to cross that threshold is not to leave behind this work of clarity about the biblical ethic. The ethic is the standard for expressing genuine compassion as we face the difficult circumstances of human experience. It is like using a plumb line to build an edifice that will not fall over.

The church's doctrines of God's sovereignty and our belonging to God and to the body of believers are reaffirmed every time a baby is presented for dedication or baptism and every time we partake of the Lord's Supper. The special commitment to each new baby is the church's affirmation that every child belongs to us as a gift from God, and we pledge ourselves to nurture and care for each child. Baptism affirms the promise of Christ's redemption of us, the promise of our adoption into the family of God, and Jesus' victory over the circumstances of life. The church has no ritual of deciding which child belongs and which child is a mistake, or unwanted.

The corporate vows we take can be a rich underpinning for the church's pastoral ministry of affirming the value of every child. Raising children in the nurture and admonition of the Lord with the support of the body should lead the local church to look with care at the needs of families within its own congregation and in the community. This admonition should extend to both opportunities to meet physical needs, as well as teaching opportunities.

What is signified by baptism and the Lord's Supper lead the church very naturally to affirm and promote the adoption of children into Christian families as a life-giving alternative to abortion. Adoption is still too neglected an area of involvement for the church. The reality of the situation *Roe* created is that the demand far exceeds the supply of babies available for adoption. The church has not yet entered this area of ministry effectively. Some couples spend many thousands of dollars on adoption hopes that never materialize. Church members and church structures include all the gifts and abilities and resources to make an overwhelming difference in uniting couples and needy children, and to turn abortions into adoptions.

Forgiveness and Restoration

Central in the doctrines of the church and signified in the Lord's Supper is the life-restoring message of the gospel: forgiveness and restoration. The

255

statement of the Presbyterian Church in 1869 that so dramatically warned those guilty of abortion that "except they repent, they cannot inherit eternal life" did no more and no less than speak the gospel to this particular sin of abortion, and point the way to redemption that is the only way of escape from any sin. Their statement may sound harsh to our ears, but consider the sort of compassion today that says nothing at all about abortion, so that women especially are thereby encouraged to believe either that it is not a sin or, conversely, that it is an unspeakable sin for which there is no remedy.

An example of compassion disconnected from the biblical ethic comes from the testimony of a clergywoman who tells the story of being contacted by a school nurse about a fifteen-year-old girl who was in her office, pregnant and in distress. The girl was afraid to tell her father for fear of punishment. Avoiding contact with the family, the clergywoman drove to the school, picked up the young girl and drove her to an abortion facility, talking to her on the way about the girl's hopes and dreams for the future. After the abortion, the clergywoman drove her back to school and delivered her, according to her own account, into the hands of a public school professional — not her own family — to deal with the aftermath of the abortion. Then she drove away. That is all she ever knew about the young girl, and she never met the girl's parents. She testifies to this experience as an example of her effort to provide compassionate support to young pregnant women.[12]

The ministry of the church that emerges from its own doctrines should be very different from this sort of compassion. The church's message is God's intervention in history and in our lives in order to change the way things are: to heal us, to save us, to forgive us, to restore us, to comfort and redeem us. The sin of abortion must not be left outside that message. This aspect of the church's ministry preserves and proclaims the truth, and speaks into the culture with the biblical norm, the Christian standards for living, and the way of escape from our own sinfulness.

In an article entitled "The Dilemmas of a Pro-Life Pastor"[13] Frederica Mathewes-Green discusses the difficulties for pastors who are clear about the standard, but feel quite alone in applying it. The article presents a series of sit-

---

12. Based on testimony from the Reverend Dr. Katherine Hancock Radgsdale, Episcopal Priest and Chair of the Board of the Religious Coalition for Reproductive Choice before the House Judiciary Committee, Subcommittee on the Constitution, The Child Custody Protection Act H.R., 3682/S. 1645, May 21, 1998 (http://www.rcrc.org/current/testimony.html, 2/19/99), 1.

13. Frederica Mathewes-Green, "The Dilemmas of a Pro-Life Pastor," *Christianity Today,* April 7, 1997, pp. 27-31.

uations fraught with moral overtones to demonstrate how difficult it is to provide good pastoral care in the face of prevailing cultural norms.

The first situation involves a pastor faced with a request from a young single mother to have him baptize her baby in his church. The second case is a pastor's dilemma of how to treat an unmarried pregnant woman in the congregation. He wants to show loving care without affirming the sinful behavior that led to the pregnancy, and he doesn't want to convey to others that the sin is being overlooked. In a third situation, a pastor who knows there are women in his congregation who have had abortions is afraid to preach on the subject for fear of offending those women or for fear of producing other kinds of emotional outbursts. Each of the situations shows the complexity of applying the biblical ethic to pastoral care in real life situations.

Pastoral care is difficult in these situations for a couple of reasons. First of all, there is too little theological thinking and discussion of abortion in our day, and a consequent ambiguity and lack of agreement about the church's ethical standard, particularly when the culture appears to accept immorality as normative behavior. Second, it is difficult even for those who are clear about the ethical standard because pastoral care lies within the disciplinary role of the church. It does not take abortion to bring out the modern church's aversion to discipline. One writer vividly compared church discipline to a root canal, antithetical to modern society's dictum that all opinions are equally valid.[14] A recovery of the biblical understanding and practice of discipline, however, is necessary to providing pastoral care that leads people toward decisions that please God and ministers restoration to those who have fallen. The Second Helvetic Confession underscores the church's long-standing attitude toward the positive role of discipline:

> . . . Since discipline is an absolute necessity in the church, it also falls to ministers to regulate this discipline for edification. . . . At all times and in all places the rule is to be observed that everything is to be done for edification, decently and honorably, without oppression and strife. For the apostle testifies that authority in the Church was given to him by the Lord for building up and not for destroying (2 Cor. 10:8).[15]

14. Tom Price, "Church Discipline and Reconciliation," *The Christian Century,* July 29–Aug. 5, 1992, pp. 702-3.

15. "Of the Ministers of the Church, Their Institution and Duties," *The Second Helvetic Confession* (Chapter XVIII). The confession was written by Heinrich Bullinger, successor to Ulrich Zwingli in Zurich, and adopted by the churches of Switzerland as their confession of faith in the mid-sixteenth century. This statement appears near the close of the chapter cited.

The goal of church discipline is discipleship. The purpose is to produce a renewed and unified body, pleasing to God and productive for his kingdom. The church exercises discipline in order to preserve sound doctrine within its borders and to protect its people from sin. Further, church discipline is the means of reclaiming those who fall away. It is the church's calling to go after the one who has strayed from the ninety and nine and bring that sheep back into the fold. Jesus ends the parable by saying, "Just so, I tell you, there will be more joy in heaven over one sinner who repents than over ninety-nine righteous persons who need no repentance" (Luke 15:4-7). And so is the joy in heaven over every person restored after abortion. We dare not forget that is what the gospel message is about. The New Testament author of Hebrews writes that "For the moment all discipline seems painful rather than pleasant; later it yields the peaceful fruit of righteousness to those who have been trained by it" (Heb. 12:11).

In a very typical mainline church in Virginia not long ago, the pastor's youngest daughter, a high-school sophomore, became pregnant. She went to her parents, frightened and filled with remorse. After absorbing the shock and after a long talk with their daughter, and fighting their own overwhelming sense of shame, the parents asked her if she would submit herself to the session of the church for spiritual guidance. She was a member of the church, as was the father of the child, although she would not name him and he did not come forward with her. After a difficult personal struggle, the young woman agreed. The session, for their part, was more taken aback by the pastor's suggestion than the teenager. They had never before been called upon to exercise their disciplinary role in this or any other respect, and they found themselves completely unprepared. Nevertheless, they agreed.

The outcome was a miracle of God's grace. Session members met with, counseled, prayed with, and helped the young woman through the decisions she had to make about her own and her baby's futures. She had already sought the forgiveness of God and her parents; the session helped her to confirm her repentance through actions that led her to restored relationships. The young father, watching from a distance, came to desire the same difficult blessing in his own life. He surprised the session by coming to the elders later with his own confession and desire for help. This was the church learning to exercise its disciplinary role in the restoration of two young lives.

Formulating Pastoral Care Strategies
through Leadership Discussions

There are few models for pastoral care in our modern church. The Mathewes-Green article shows that rather ordinary situations can become overwhelming moral dilemmas in a church that has become accustomed to silence on abortion. It is worth some emotional cost among church leaders to devote time to preparing themselves spiritually with the rudiments of a plan for how they will respond corporately to situations that exist and might arise in their own congregations. The following questions are among those that might be considered. How would we in the church apply the biblical ethic to these situations? What practical options for action might we consider that would be faithful expressions of our Christian faith? Look at the people and the resources in the congregation and consider how the church should respond:

- to a young couple when they learn they are faced with a high-risk pregnancy, and are being counseled to consider abortion;
- to a family that learns of the pregnancy of their fifteen-year-old daughter;
- to a high-school youth who reveals that his girlfriend is pregnant just as he is preparing to leave for college;
- to a young single woman who appears in church with her child born out of wedlock;
- to a childless couple when they decide to consider adoption.

Pastor Gary LeTourneau says that capitulating to the notion that abortion is too divisive an issue to deal with in the church produces four losers. The first is the unborn babies, who continue to die even at the hands of their Christian mothers. Then there are the mothers, who are never warned prior to their sin and never have the opportunity to repent and be restored following an abortion. Another loser is the church, which experiences the pollution of repeated and unconfessed sin by its members. And last, but not least, is the minister, who certainly feels guilty, and who is guilty of the sin of silence in the face of the slaughter of innocent victims.[16]

Women who are pregnant and, for whatever the reason, are considering abortion as a solution, are often women facing adverse circumstances. The

---

16. Gary LeTourneau, "Abortion and Church Discipline," unpublished manuscript of paper presented at a consultation on the Church and Abortion, Princeton Seminary, 1992.

abortion is evidence that they are in a search for help for a solution. Pastors and church members who fear the terrible consequences of a commitment to speak to and minister to these situations are also facing adversity and, just like those women, are facing a spiritual challenge. The church needs to pray that pastors and other believers will meet the challenge faithfully, for their own sakes, for the sakes of the mothers, and for the sakes of unborn children.

Index

Centre for Bioethics and Public Policy, 78

Chlamydia, 84-85

Christianity Today, 166

Christian Medical & Dental Society (CMDS), 170, 177n.8, 178-79

Christian mind, 213-25

The Christian Mind: How Should a Christian Think? (Harry Blamires), 213

Christians: in academia, 91-93, 97; and bioethics, 221, 233-34; difference of faith for, 4-5; and the disabled, 203, 205; divisions among, 5-6, 12, 33-34, 60; in health care, 171-74, 179, 181-85; and the media, 15, 101-10; and politics, 5-9, 10-14; in postmodern world, 222-24, 225, 227-34

Christian professional networks, 75-76

church, 76-77, 211-19, 231-32; and abortion, 250-60; and bioethics, 226-27, 230; and the disabled, 199-200, 201-2; and discipline, 257-58; and quietism, 242; and social justice, 237

Clinton, Bill, 104-5, 137, 149n.6

Coalition for Urgent Research (CURE), 166

Coalition of Americans for Research Ethics (CARE), 165

Code of Ethics (Social Work), 41, 43, 44, 49-50, 51-52, 54

colleges and universities: Christian, 73-75, 90, 93; Christian challenges within, 95-97; Christian silence within, 89, 91-92; secular, 89-90, 91-93

Colson, Charles, 186

compromise, 8-9, 243

condoms, 83, 84-85

confession, 66

Confession of 1967, 237

Congressional Ethics Committee, 133, 136-37

Congressional Office of Technology Assessment (OTA), 137-38

Constitution, 147-48

"constitutional rights" theory, 160

core values, 41, 46, 49-50

Creamer, Deborah, 200

"Crimes and Misdemeanors" (Woody Allen film), 187, 190

cryopreservation, 151-63

cynicism, 14

Darwin's Black Box (Michael Behe), 194

David, 58-62

Davis v. Davis, 156-57n.20, 161-62, 164

deconstructionism, 189

Del Zios v. Columbia Presbyterian Medical Center, 155

Department of Health, Education and Welfare, 134, 136

Department of Health and Human Services (DHHS), 132-33, 135, 136, 149n.6. *See also* Department of Health, Education and Welfare

dialysis rationing, 192

disability, 196, 197-99; and the church, 199-200, 201-2; pain of, 204; and spiritual needs, 202-3; supporting those with, 206-8

discipleship, 258

"Do No Harm," 165

Door of Hope, 246

Dossey, Larry, 63-64

Dworkin, Ronald, 218

Elders, Jocelyn, 82

Elijah, 66

embryo transfer, 135

Epaphroditus, 67

epidictic discourse, 239

Esther, 183-85

ethical dilemmas, 43-44

ethics, 40-56; autonomy, 25, 27; professional, 37-38, 41-44, 54-56; social, 236-41. *See also* utilitarianism

Ethics Advisory Board, 132, 135-36

euthanasia, 174-75; Michigan campaign against, 174, 178-79

Evangelium Vitae (John Paul II), 249

evolution, 123-24

faith, 33

fallenness, 48